BASIC

pilates

Susanne Barry

MQP

About the author

Susanne Barry dedicates herself to bringing her lifelong passion and holistic approach to health and well-being to others. Her work has included children's fitness, fitness for the over-fifties, specialist cardiac rehabilitation instruction, and working with medical practitioners to set up exercise classes for their patients. She holds a degree in psychology and is a certified hypnotherapist. Susanne specializes in Pilates and lives and teaches in Hertfordshire, England.

Acknowledgments

I would like to thank all my students, from whom I have learned so much. Andrew Harwich, my osteopath, for releasing me from back pain and introducing me to Pilates. Andi Vincent Jones, for encouraging my body to go where I thought it couldn't, and Coleen at Redbourn physiotherapy clinic.

To Carolyn Free Pearce for herself. To Body Control Pilates for their teacher training and excellent professional development.

And to the models—Maria, Shelley, and Craig.

Caution

If you are pregnant, have given birth in the last six weeks, or have a medical condition, such as high blood pressure, spinal problems, arthritis, or asthma, consult your medical practitioner or an experienced teacher before any exercise.

Published by MQ Publications Limited
12 The Ivories
6–8 Northampton Street
London N1 2HY
Tel: 020 7359 2244
Fax: 020 7359 1616
Email: mail@mqpublications.com
Website: www.mqpublications.com

Editor: Abi Rowsell
Design: Balley Design Associates
Illustrations: Oxford Designers & Illustrators
Photography: Stuart Boreham

ISBN: 1-84072-497-8
1 3 5 7 9 0 8 6 4 2

Printed in China

contents

foreword

"I cannot teach you ... only help you to explore yourself, nothing more." Bruce Lee

Pilates is a journey of self-awareness, linking the mind, body, and senses. It encompasses the physical, emotional, cognitive, and spiritual aspects of our being. It's about making time for ourselves on a regular basis, and listening to what our bodies have to say. It is not, however, a quick-fix solution. It is a journey of discovery, a way of learning to stop and listen, to be present with your body. This takes time, practice, and effort. When you first look at the exercises they seem quite simple—but simple doesn't mean easy!

Physical symptoms can often be a manifestation of what's going on in your life. Pain is the body's way of telling us that something is not working. How often do you get tight shoulders or a pain in the neck? Could that be linked to the people you are with or the job that you do? We may even say that someone or something is "a pain in the neck!" It's understandable that sometimes we don't listen to these warning signs, because to listen might mean that we need to change and move out of our "comfort zone." That's why we sometimes "choose" to live with the pain in the neck. But if you want to take responsibility for your own health and well-being, reading this book can be a first step, and you may find it's one of the best decisions you ever made.

Pilates is different from any other exercise system. Now one of the most popular exercise systems, it was invented by the German Joseph Pilates (1880–1967), a very determined individual with multiple problems. With extraordinary dedication, he worked on his body until he was an accomplished athlete, capable of body building, skiing, gymnastics, dance, yoga, and boxing, amongst other skills. Not content to follow traditional fitness regimes, he developed his own method, drawing from the various disciplines that he had practiced to build strength, flexibility, balance, and coordination, and incorporating a fusion of Eastern and Western ideals.

Pilates involves a quality of awareness that extends way beyond the body. Because it is so different, it takes time to adjust. Be patient, persevere, be interested, be curious, and be excited to learn about your own amazing body. Even after you have been doing a certain exercise for many months, you may suddenly feel or experience it in a slightly different way because your body is changing.

Pilates works from the inside out, targeting deep postural muscles to give you strength, balance, coordination, and poise—not forgetting, of course, that elusive flat stomach, tight butt, and overall muscle tone. The great thing about it is that all you need for a Pilates work-out is you and a space. It is the ultimate portable "gym" that everyone can do, from complete beginners to professional athletes.

The real aim of this book is to enable you to become your own teacher and guide. Yes, it would help if you could also attend classes, but mainly I hope that after trying Pilates, you will feel more comfortable in your own body, whatever its shape or size, or level of ability. To move with grace and ease, to enjoy movement and your body—that is what is important.

Susanne Barry

introduction

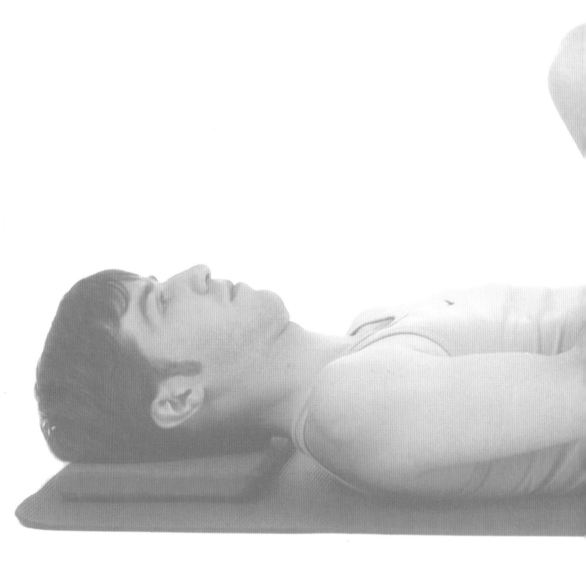

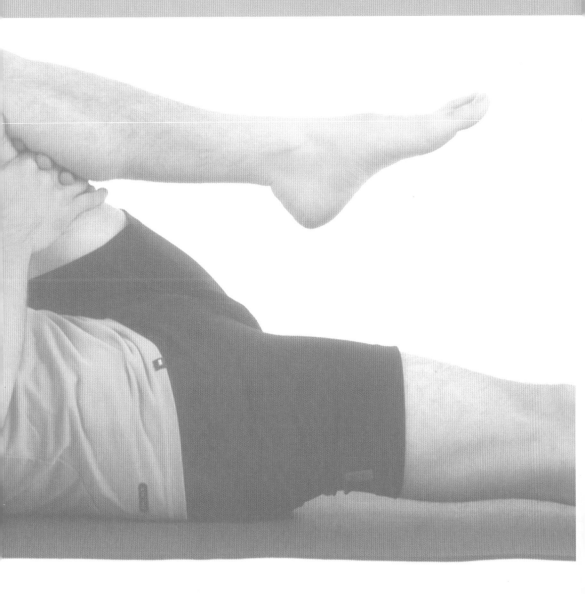

how to use this book

This book is designed so that you can start with the Principles of Pilates and work your way through, progressing to the next stage when you are ready. The exercises are divided into The Warm-up, followed by three stages—Starting Off, Moving On, and Intermediate. Each stage is a workout on its own. For shorter workouts, you can follow either the 20- or 45-minute programs for each stage at the back of the book.

It is important to practice the Principles, but it may take a while before they feel natural and automatic. That's fine—just keep practicing. The Warm-up is designed to prepare your spine for activity. It provides a basic workout that includes all the elements you need to keep your spine healthy, so if you are short of time, or don't want to think too much about which exercises to do, the Warm-up is a complete workout in itself. Practice the exercises in the Warm-up before you move on to the next stage. How quickly you progress through the book will depend on your current health and fitness levels and how often you practice.

functions of the exercises

You will see the functions highlighted under the heading of each exercise. If there are specific preparations for an exercise, this will also be mentioned uner the heading.

■ **Release**—this provides a stretch or release for a certain area (or areas) of the body.

■ **Stability**—this uses the abdominals or other stabilizing muscles to keep the trunk still while you are moving. Some exercises may have more than one function; for example, Shoulder Release on page 68 helps to release the chest and shoulder muscles but you will also be working to stabilize the trunk with your abdominal and upper back muscles.

■ **Flexion**—this means bending. One of the fundamentals in Pilates is to learn to move your spine like a wheel. It's easy to achieve in the thoracic (mid-back) area, but a lumbar (lower back) curve is more difficult because you need strong abdominal muscles to initiate this movement. You will be practicing this in Spine Curl (see page 50).

■ **Rotation**—this is a turning movement of the trunk. Imagine twisting as if you're putting a seat belt on. Rotation needs to be practiced or the mobility can be lost.

■ **Extension**—this is the opposite of flexion, in other words "straightening." Extension is an important movement to practice as the force of gravity is always pushing us toward a flexed position—that's one of the reasons why it's so hard to sit and stand straight. An example of an extension exercise is the Upper Back Press (see page 58).

Each type of movement is important. You may find some movements easier than others, in which case you should make a note as you work through. Are your favorite exercises mainly flexion, rotation, or extension?

Once you have worked through all the sections in the book, you will be able to compile your own workouts. Understanding the functions of each of the exercises will help you to compile your workout with exercises from the different stages, ensuring you include a balance of each of the functions.

making pilates a habit

Pilates doesn't have to be another "should" or "to do" on your list, just decide to make Pilates part of your life and work toward that goal. There is no need to rush through the exercises to improve, or progress; enjoy the improvements in the quality of your life now.

Making time for yourself can be hard, especially if you have a busy job or a family to care for—or both. But as you start to make time for yourself on a regular basis you will find that you look forward to your Pilates sessions. Being totally immersed in an activity, has such a transformational effect on mood and health that you will find you don't have to "plan" or "make time" any more, because it will become as natural as cleaning your teeth.

If you've had a negative view of exercise in the past, then reframe it. Look at it from a different point of view; "see" yourself differently, visualize yourself performing the movements with ease; believe that you can.

Health advice

Don't exercise if you are over-tired or unwell. If any movement or exercise causes you pain, stop immediately; if the pain persists, consult your physician. Pilates is not an aerobic exercise (i.e. one that provides cardiovascular benefits). It's a good idea to complement Pilates with walking or jogging, cycling, dancing, or any other activities that raise your heart rate for a sustained period.

Before embarking on any exercise program, seek medical advice, particularly if you have current health issues, suffer from chronic pain, have sustained injuries, or if you are pregnant.

what you will need

- A mat or folded blanket, 1 to 2 inches thick
- A hand towel or paperback book to rest your head on
- A hand towel or firm pillow, in case you need to modify any exercises
- Comfortable clothes that won't restrict your movement. You may want to choose close-fitting garments so you can observe your body.
- A warm room
- Relaxing music
- Scented candles (optional)
- Freedom from distractions. Turn off the phone and, if you share your home with others, ask them not to disturb you.

Joseph Pilates recommended that you exercise four times weekly for a period of 15 to 30 minutes per session. You will find what works for you, and which times are best for you. Some people prefer getting up slightly earlier while others like to practice after work. Sometimes I think "I've got to much to do, I'm too tired. I'll just come down to my mat for a 10-minute relaxation." But once I've relaxed and practiced some deep breathing, I feel better and start to do a couple of exercises, and before I know it an hour and a half has passed! I feel great, completely re-energized, with my mood transformed. It's the next best thing to great sex I know of.

So the next time you hear yourself saying "I haven't got time," why not just get started and go with the flow?

mind/body together

"Nothing holds more power over the body than the beliefs of the mind."

Deepak Chopra, *Ageless Body, Timeless Mind*

It's very important what people think about while they are doing Pilates. Pilates is precise. It's essential to have correct alignment so that the correct muscles are used, but "precise" does not mean "perfect." If you try too hard you will soon get tense—and the idea is that you should be releasing muscle tension before you move. Gaining confidence in your body and movement will come as you develop your awareness. If you feel discouraged about how long it is taking, celebrate the fact that you are on the path. If you find yourself worrying that you aren't doing it right, take your awareness back into your body and repeat the following affirmations: "I feel my muscles releasing, expressing their joy of moving;" "I can see myself doing my exercises with ease;" "I am grateful to have this time, and my current levels of health and vitality." Affirmations are a powerful means of reframing the way you perceive something. Or ask yourself these questions to develop your awareness: "Where are my feet in relation to my knees? Where are my knees in relation to my hips? Am I straight along my mat? Where are my eyes focused? Where do I store tension in my body? In what part of my body do I feel this exercise?" Let your body be your teacher. Bring what is unconscious into consciousness and remember—"precise" doesn't mean "perfect."

The meditative qualities of Pilates help you to become more aware of how you feel, providing a link to your emotions. Even if you think you haven't got time to do any exercises, just by starting with the breathing exercises and becoming aware of your body, you will develop greater insight. Awareness of how emotions or feelings are manifested in your body are the first steps toward recognizing them, acknowledging them, understanding them, and choosing whether or not you want to express these emotions in this way.

Fear and anger are often portrayed as "negative emotions." Although they may manifest themselves negatively in modern life, they are not negative per se—they are vital for our survival, so respect them, listen to them in your body, and learn what they have to teach you, before they shout at you with illness. Where do emotions go in your body? Chronic backache, or tightness in the chest, aching shoulders and neck, stiff joints, chest complaints? Even if you don't have time to do a Pilates workout every time you feel stressed, you can just breathe and stop to let yourself become aware. Slow down and come back to your body. You can do this anywhere, and create a feeling of calm within you at any time, once you take your awareness into your body. How we feel emotionally is directly related to what's happening in our body, and the understanding of this is what makes Pilates so much more than an exercise method. Once you start to link responses in your body to what's happening in your life, it is very empowering. Start now by practicing the habit of relaxation instead of the habit of stress. (For breathing awareness, see page 28.)

Remember: Your body cannot tell the difference between a real or imagined experience. Use your imagination creatively and be kind to yourself.

postural habits

Alignment is one of the key principles of Pilates, and learning about your alignment will help to improve your posture. You only have to look at how the majority of our time is spent to see that the life we live is reflected in our bodies. We start early, hunched over desks at school, then move on to computers, sitting in cars, and leading sedentary lives. Some occupations require that we work in awkward positions—musicians, dentists, and nurses are good examples of this. Sports that favor one side, such as golf or tennis, create imbalances of strength and flexibility. In normal fitness workouts, muscular imbalances are exaggerated—weak muscles get weaker and strong muscles get stronger. Pilates works to bring balance back to the body; its holistic approach ensures that your whole body is involved, from your brain to your feet.

It's not only lifestyle that has an effect on posture. Your posture will also be influenced—but not determined—by your genes. If you want to know what you will look like in a few years—without Pilates, of course!—look at your parents. Who are you most like?

The skeleton and joints are unlikely to be changed by Pilates, but posture is improved because Pilates balances the way the muscles and tendons exert force on the bones. You will see improvements relatively quickly after doing just a few simple exercises and by developing an awareness during your everyday life. This will help ensure that the benefits of the exercises are transferred to what you do, day in, day out.

The ideal posture shown on page 20 may be rare in everyday life, but it is a great goal to work toward. An ideal posture is one in which the body can function most efficiently, with the least effort. That means the minimum of work for your muscles and joints. Although the typical slouched posture of a teenager creates less work for the muscles, it places more stress or load on the joints. When the teenager slouches, over a period of time adaptive changes take place. For instance, one or two vertebrae in the spine may become less

mobile, and this change will affect the neighboring vertebrae as they will need to become more mobile to make up for the restricted areas. In this way, the stiff areas get stiffer while the mobile areas get used more to compensate.

Improving posture requires a combination of elements: Awareness of where your body is now, identifying the areas that need to be stretched and those which need to be strengthened, and practicing new postural habits. We can start to change the way we move by thinking of our postures as habits—postural habits. A habit is something that has been acquired with many repetitions over a period of time. The good thing about habits is that they can be broken. It takes thousands of repetitions to program a movement or behavior into the nervous system so that it becomes automatic. That's why it also takes time to unlearn them. When you start Pilates, you may get frustrated if you don't see instant results or attain perfect posture immediately, but you have to wait for your body to become structurally different—stronger in some areas, more flexible in others—before you can hold good posture with the minimum of effort. The key is to keep practicing.

chapter 2

principles of pilates

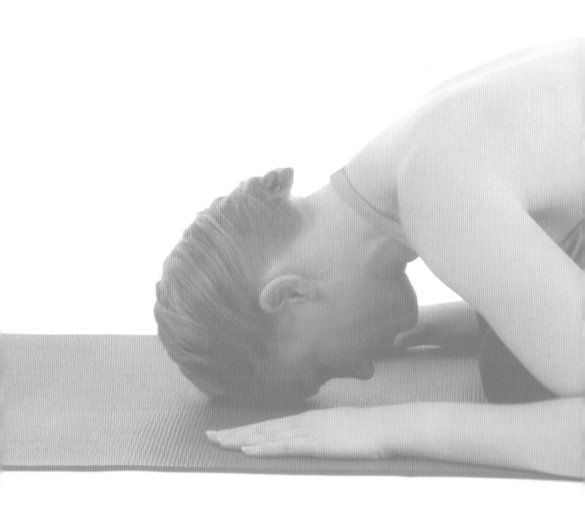

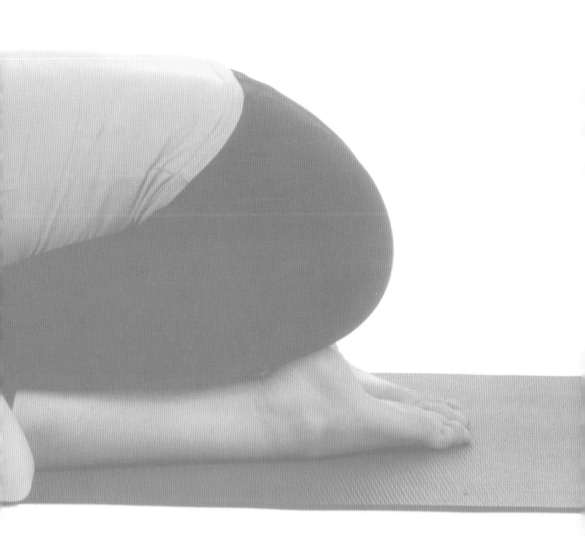

- relaxation and awareness
- precision and alignment
- breathing
- stabilizing or centering

relaxation and awareness

The essential principles to consider when you are practicing Pilates are Relaxation (or release), Awareness, Precision and Alignment, Breathing, Stabilizing, Coordination and Balance, Flowing Movements, Endurance, and, importantly, Regular Practice. The principles of relaxation and awareness are dependent on each other. How can you begin to release tight muscles if you are not aware of them? By becoming aware of your body, you will start to develop a sense of where you feel tension and need to release. It is a physical and psychological preparation, a way of letting go of stresses and tensions from your mind and body. Mindfulness is a large part of what you will be cultivating in Pilates, training both the mind and the body, focusing your mind on every part of the movement, developing your kinesthetic awareness of where your body is in space and time.

relaxation position

The Relaxation Position is the starting position for many Pilates exercises and is also a good position in which to spend a few minutes at the start of your session. Come down to your mat and lie in this position, taking your awareness to different parts of your body to see where there is tension. This body scan can take as little as a minute or as long as 20—it depends on how how much time you feel you need to bring balance to your body.

1 Sit on the floor with your knees bent, feet on the floor. Gently roll over onto your side and rest your head on a paperback book or a folded towel.

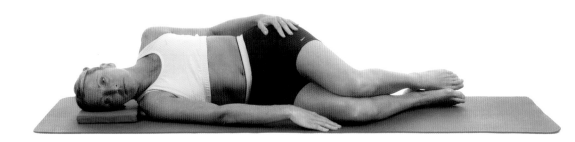

2 Keeping your head down, roll over onto your back. Reposition the book or towel under your head. This way of coming down to your mat is especially helpful if you suffer from back or neck problems.

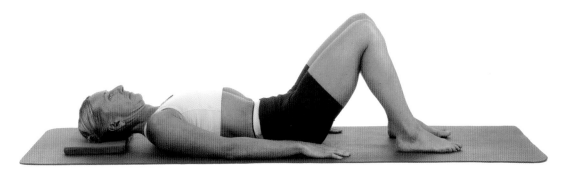

3 Your knees are bent and slightly apart, in line with your hip bones. Position your feet firmly on the floor, lining them up with your hip bones and knees. Check that you are lying straight on your mat.

4 Let the back of your head sink down into the floor or book. Keep the back of your neck long. Take a deep breath in and, as you exhale, let go of any tension between your eyebrows. Take another deep breath in and, as you breathe out, release any tension in your jaw. As you become aware of the heaviness of your head, you will feel your neck and shoulder muscles release, dropping heavier into the mat. Your arms feel heavy and this feeling of release spreads out along the collar bones and chest, and you sense a widening in your chest and upper back.

5 Take another deep breath and, as you breathe out, let your bottom and hips sink down into the mat so the muscles at the front of the hips and lower back release. Think about the weight that is being supported in your feet. The next time you take a deep breath, imagine you are directing your breath all the way into your fingers and toes, and let go of any tension with the out breath.

precision and alignment

Correct alignment is essential to ensure that the right muscle groups are being used and balance is being restored to your body. A good way to become aware of posture is to exaggerate a bad posture and imagine what the cumulative effects would be over time. Round your upper back and notice what happens to your line of sight—you will be looking slightly down. To see properly, you would have to create a greater curvature, and thus strain, in the neck. This is a common posture in many elderly (and not so elderly!) people.

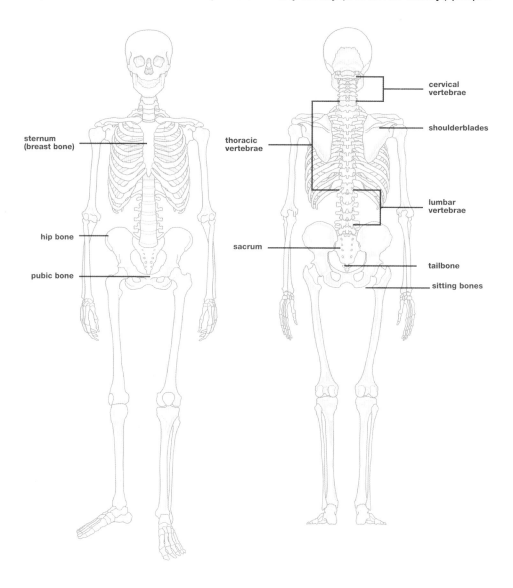

sternum
(breast bone)

hip bone

pubic bone

thoracic
vertebrae

sacrum

cervical
vertebrae

shoulderblades

lumbar
vertebrae

tailbone

sitting bones

ideal posture

A good way of thinking about how your body is aligned is to imagine a plumbline passing through your body. It falls through the ear and the vertebrae of the neck, the front of the shoulder, ribs, lumbar vertebrae, slightly behind the hip joint, just in front of the center of the knee, and just in front of the ankle bone. Compare where the plumbline falls in an ideal posture with its position in the two kinds of postural imbalances shown below.

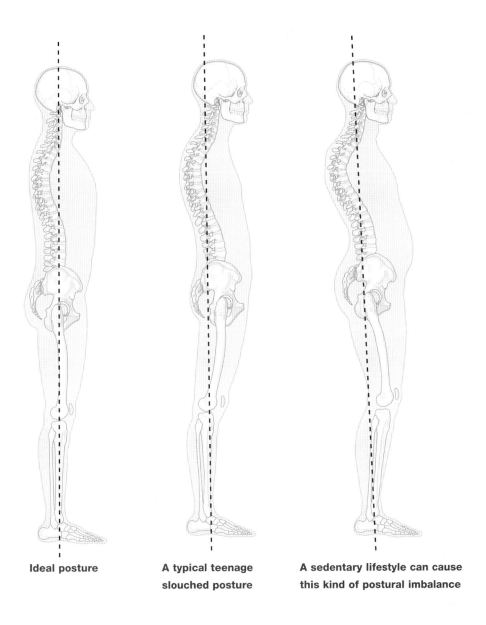

Ideal posture

A typical teenage slouched posture

A sedentary lifestyle can cause this kind of postural imbalance

correct alignment when standing

1 To find a good standing posture, start with your feet about hip distance apart, either parallel or slightly turned out. In the turned-out position, used for some exercises, the heels are closer together than the toes. Your knees are in line with your feet, and they should be "soft"—this means straight but not "locked."

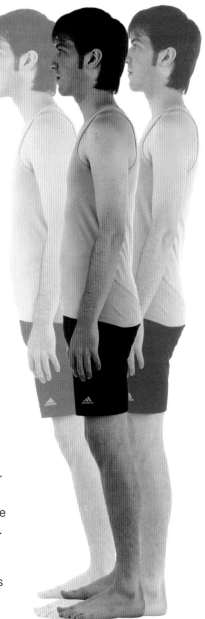

2 Think about where your weight is balanced in your feet. Do you carry your weight mainly in your toes, or heels, or is it spread evenly? Start to rock very gently, as if you're being blown by the wind, until you feel slightly more weight in your toes while keeping your heels on the ground. Then reverse, so that there is slightly more weight in your heels, keeping your toes down. Did you notice anything else happening as you were doing this? Perhaps you felt a tightening in your buttocks, abdominal muscles, or back. This is an example of your postural muscles working to keep you standing upright.

3 Focus on your right foot and leg. Do you hold more weight on one side of the body than the other? Gently sway side to side, feeling the weight being transferred to the outsides and insides of your feet. Then think about spreading the weight evenly between the base of the big toe, the base of little toe and the center of the heel, in the shape of a triangle. Your feet shouldn't roll in nor out. Visualize a lengthening up through your spine. Lift the crown of the head up as you gently draw your shoulderblades down your back. Let your head go forward and up, neck long and eyes focused at eye level.

bending knees

How well the arches in your feet support you is important in foot, knee, and hip alignment. Flat feet will contribute to back or neck problems. Do this exercise to improve alignment and to work the foot muscles that support the arches in your feet.

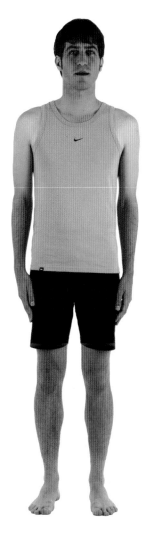

1 Stand with your feet parallel and lightly squeeze the backs of your inner thighs together as you bend your knees over your toes, aiming the middle of the kneecap toward your second toe. Keep squeezing the backs of your inner thighs together as you bend your knees. Don't let the inside of either foot roll toward the other.

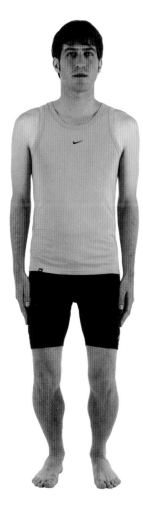

2 Straighten your legs, still squeezing the backs of your inner thighs together. Can you feel that the action of bringing the back of the inner thighs together starts to lift and work the muscles that support the arches in your feet? Repeat 6 to 10 times.

neutral sitting position

The aim in Pilates is to work with the spine following its natural curves. To do this, we have to learn how to stabilize the pelvis in a neutral position, halfway between full flexion and full extension, so that your pubic bone and your hip bones are level.

The first photograph (a) shows a common sitting position, with a slumped lower back. Can you see how the tailbone is tucked under and the normal lumbar curve has been lost? If we didn't have such comfortable chairs, it would be very uncomfortable to roll back with the weight on the tailbone like this.

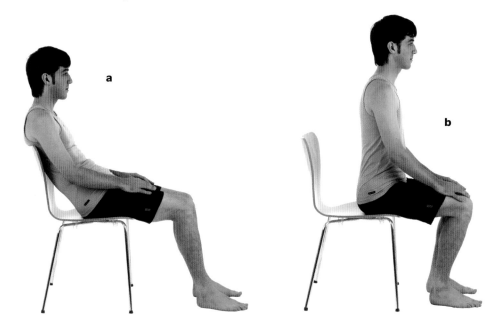

In a good sitting position (b), you will be further forward on the chair with your weight equally placed in the center of your sitting bones in your buttocks. Your legs should be bent at right angles to your hips, about shoulder-width apart. Bend your knees at right angles and place your feet firmly on the floor to help support your weight. Think about a plumbline running through your ear, the tip of your shoulder and your hip. Imagine that the top of your head is floating upward, lengthening the spine, and creating space between each vertebra. Imagine your tailbone dropping down as if it were resting on the chair behind you.

progression—sofa stretch

If you are seated for most of the day, your hamstring muscles (at the back of your legs) will be tight. Maybe you usually come home and slump down on a sofa or comfy chair to relax or watch your favorite soap, but why not try the following exercise, known as Soap Stretch, instead?

1 Sit with a folded towel under your hips with your back supported by a chair or sofa and your legs straight out in front of you. Bend one knee up toward your chest or out to the side, whichever feels most comfortable. Sit up as straight as you can, so that you feel a gentle stretch or pulling in the back of your straight leg. If it feels too strong, bend the straight leg a little.
2 Change your legs every few minutes. Aim to sit like this for 5 or 10 minutes to start with, and alternate between bending your knee upward and moving your leg out to the side. Try to sit up as straight as you can.

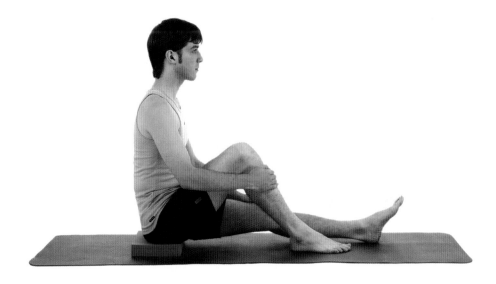

neutral standing position

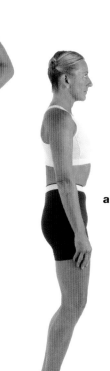

1 Stand up with good posture, as described on page 20. Place the heels of your hands on your hip bones with your fingers pointing toward your pubic bone.

2 Gently roll your tailbone under so that your pubic bone tilts upward, then release. As you roll your tailbone under you are taking your pelvis into a "posterior tilt," as shown in photograph (a).

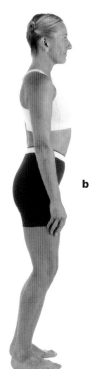

a

b

3 In photograph (b), the pelvis is in an anterior tilt, where the lumbar curve is exaggerated. Don't try this position—it's not good for your back.

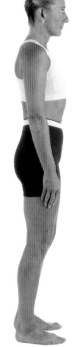

c

4 Photograph (c) shows the pelvis in a neutral position, between the other two positions. The hip bones and the pubic bone are on the same plane. This is what you are aiming at.

four point kneeling position

1 Kneel on all fours with the heels of your hands directly underneath your shoulders, and shoulder-width apart, your knees underneath your hips, hip distance apart. Look directly down in between your hands to ensure that your head is in line with your spine. Make sure that your weight is evenly distributed from the heel of your hand to your fingers and thumb, and ensure your fingers are pointing forward in line with your arms. Think of pushing the floor away from you and, as you do this, draw your shoulderblades down your back, away from your ears.

2 Now roll the pelvis as you did in Neutral Standing Position, step 1, so that the pubic bone tilts toward your navel as your tailbone tucks under.

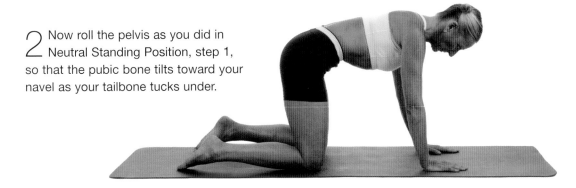

3 Roll gently the other way, just as far as feels comfortable.

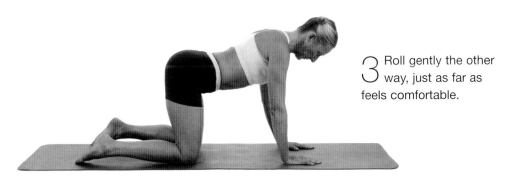

4 Find the position between steps 2 and 3 so that your tailbone isn't tucked under or tilting up. This is your neutral position. Make sure your head is in line with your spine and your neck feels comfortable.

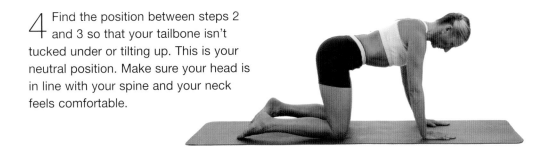

neutral in relaxation position

Finding and holding neutral is one of the most challenging parts of Pilates. Be kind to yourself if it doesn't come naturally. It took me many months to begin to feel comfortable and to be able to work from this position, and many people I teach find the same.

1 Come down to your mat as described on page 16 and make sure that your feet, knees, and hips are aligned.

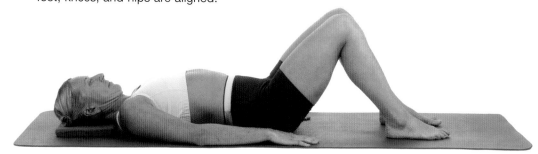

2 Gently curl your tailbone under so that your pubic bone comes toward your navel. What do you feel happening? Are your back and waist flattening into the mat? In this position the lumbar curve has been lost and your pelvis has a posterior tilt.

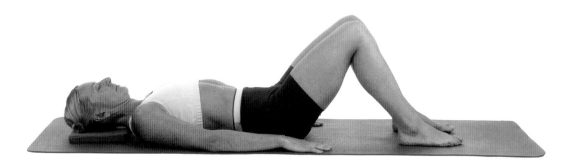

3 When the pelvis is tilted the other way (with an anterior tilt), the lower back is arched and the ribs open outward. This position is to be avoided and is shown here for demonstration only.

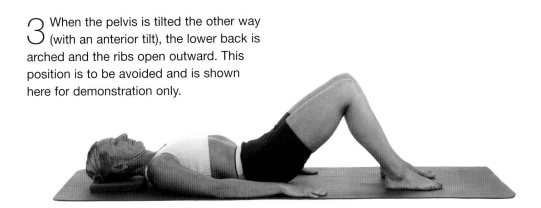

4 Neutral position is between these two positions. The hip bones and pubic bone are on the same plane. Imagine you could balance a plate with a glass of champagne there without spilling it! Or that you have a spirit level on your stomach, so that the hips bones are level from right to left. There is a natural curve in your lower back, as the tailbone lengthens away and the front of the pelvis is open.

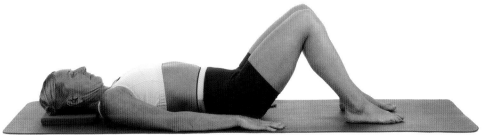

awareness

■ If the feet are too near the hips, this encourages the back to roll out of neutral into a slight posterior tilt. If the feet are too far away, the back is a little too arched. Find a comfortable position for you.

■ If you find lying in neutral uncomfortable, you can either bring your feet a little closer to your hips, which will allow the back muscles to relax a little, or place a folded towel or firm pillow under your lower back or hips, which will have the effect of rolling you slightly out of neutral and allowing the lower back to release a little. It's fine to work in this position to begin with, or if your lower back feels sore at any time, but remember that you are aiming to work without a pillow as soon as you are able. When your muscles begin to rebalance, neutral position will become more comfortable. If you find you cannot work in neutral, it might be advisable to consult a physician.

breathing

As you are reading this, start to become aware of your breath. Don't alter anything—just watch it, listen to it, and feel it in your body. Do you notice that you lengthen very slightly on the in breath and soften a little on the out breath? Can you feel any movement in your chest and shoulders, your ribs and abdominals? If you try this breathing awareness in the bath, you will find you rise out of the water on the in breath and sink down a bit on the out breath.

In Pilates we practice lateral or thoracic breathing, where we are sending the breath wide into the sides and back of the lower ribs. This is what is meant by a "wide breath." There are many benefits to expanding the ribcage in this way. It mobilizes the ribs and the muscles used in respiration, thereby increasing flexibility in the upper body. It increases lung capacity so there's more circulating oxygen to provide nourishment for organs and tissues. It can help reduce stomach acid and aids detoxification by improving the metabolism. And it promotes relaxation, thus helping to reverse the effects of the stress. This kind of deep breathing also uses the abdominal muscles, and is an excellent workout on its own.

Take a deep breath in now, and breathe out for as long as you comfortably can. Make the exhalation last. Can you feel the muscles around your trunk and abdomen working? When you practice Pilates regularly, you will develop a greater awareness of these muscles.

awareness

■ Be aware of what happens to your shoulders when you breathe. Try to watch yourself in a mirror, so you can see as well as feel the movements. With a natural breath, there is a slight extension of the body so you may notice a small movement in your shoulders, but if you constantly overuse your shoulders as you breathe, the neck and shoulder muscles will get tense and tight (as in the picture). Lateral, or thoracic breathing can help alleviate tension in these areas. If you start to feel dizzy or light-headed, only take one or two deep breaths then return to your normal breathing pattern. Think of the way a frog's sides expand and contract. Remember that it will become easier as your body adapts. In the meantime, just be patient and keep practicing.

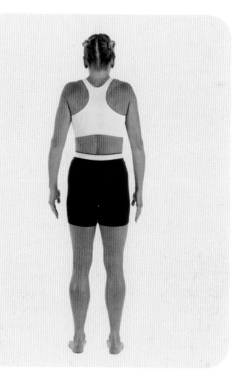

standing and breathing

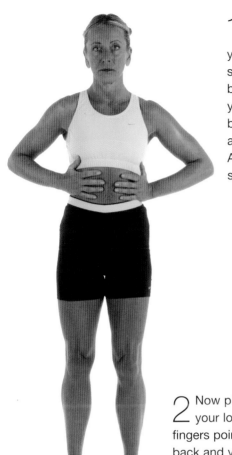

1 Stand in the good standing position described on page 20. Place your hands on your lower ribs, just above your waist. Drop your shoulders away from your ears. Take a deep breath in and think of directing the breath into your hands. Imagine your ribs expanding like bellows. Breathe out gently through your mouth, as if you are gently blowing out through a straw. As you are breathing out think of your ribs gently softening downward toward your hips.

2 Now place your hands on your lower ribs with your fingers pointing toward your back and your thumbs forward. Drop your shoulders. As you breathe in, try to feel the breath widening into your back as well as the sides of your ribs.

3 Place your hands on the front of your lower ribs, just over the diaphragm. As you breathe out, you will feel an empty space as your ribs drop down. Move your hands down your ribs as you breathe out, encouraging their natural movement. This downward movement of the ribs as you exhale is called "softening" or "closing the ribs down."

breathing in relaxation position

Wide, or lateral breathing is essential in Pilates so that you can keep your abdominal muscles working while you are moving. When you first learn the breathing technique, you will be engaging your abdominal muscles as you breathe out. Once you have mastered it, you will be able to keep the abdominals working on the in breath as well.

1 Lie down in the Relaxation Position (see page 16) with your hands by your sides (or place them on the front of your ribs to help you to feel what is happening). Breathe in to the sides and back of your ribs.

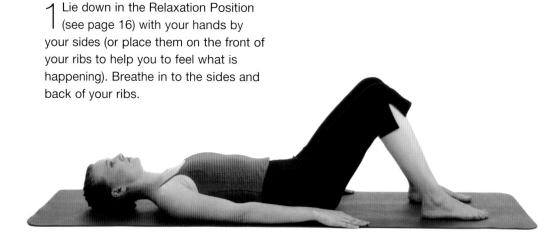

2 Breathe out and feel your ribs start to move down the front of your body. Do you feel a space under your hands now?

3 Take a "wide" breath in and feel your ribs start to expand outward. As you breathe out, feel the softening or closing down of your ribs. This is important to help keep your spine stable and to maintain the natural curves of the spine.

The normal breathing pattern is:

Breathe in—wide to the sides and back of the ribs, lengthening the spine from the crown of the head to the tailbone, preparing for movement.
Breathe out—to engage your abdominal muscles, and to move.
This pattern changes for some exercises, because the in breath aids extension (straightening), while the out breath aids flexion (bending). In some exercises, the breathing pattern will match the movement.

breathing in rest position

This is a good position in which to practice your breathing, but if you find it uncomfortable, just practice breathing in the Relaxation Position, opposite.

1 Kneel on all fours, then lower your hips back toward your heels. Slide your hands back to rest on the floor by your head or down by your sides.

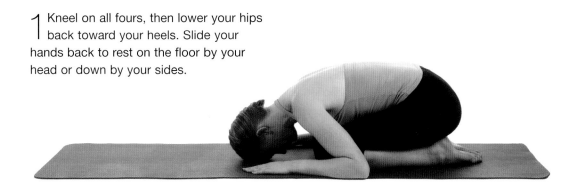

2 Follow the instructions for lateral breathing: Take a wide breath in, sending it into the sides and back of your ribs. Imagine you are directing your breath into your mid and lower back, releasing any tension there, and observing where your breath goes. Breathe out and feel the softening downward.

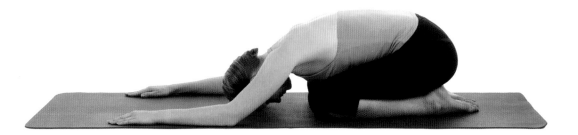

progression—breathing meditation

One meditation technique involves concentrating on your breathing. You can do this at any time, if you notice yourself becoming irritable or frustrated, or if you just want to center yourself. Sit down and close your eyes for two to three minutes and concentrate on your breathing. This is a way of slowing down and experiencing the peace of a quiet mind. What happened? Did you find any thoughts creeping in, any shoulds, or musts? If you practice this regularly, you will find that you can use it to bring a feeling of calmness into your day.

stabilizing or centering

Joseph Pilates talked about working from a strong "center" or "power house." Pilates exercises start with these power house muscles of the abdominals, lower back, hips, inner thighs, and buttocks. They enable us to stabilize the trunk, acting like your own internal corset. Think of these muscles as your foundation for movement—just as the foundations of a house keep the house stable, so the muscles of your center have to keep you stable. The muscles we are concentrating on for the next few exercises are the pelvic floor and the deep abdominal muscles (transversus abdominus). These muscles are active in everyday life, they help keep us balanced, and they are used whenever we laugh or cough. Try it now. Place one hand on your lower abdomen and the other by one of your hip bones, and cough. Did you feel the muscles contract, becoming firmer under your hands? Laughing is also an excellent workout for the deep abdominals. In Pilates, we engage these muscles (in other words, get them to work) by drawing our navel back toward our spine.

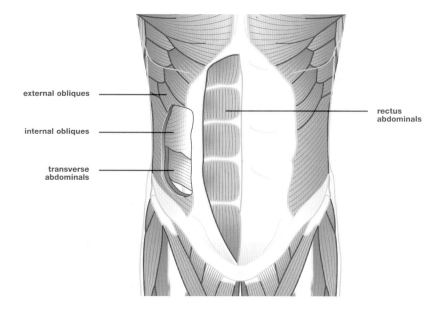

external obliques

internal obliques

transverse abdominals

rectus abdominals

engaging the pelvic floor

The pelvic floor muscles work in tandem with the transversus abdominus and they have a stabilizing function. It is important to learn awareness of these muscles and how to work them. You will be working your pelvic floor muscles in every Pilates exercise.

1 Sit in a chair, in the sitting position described on page 22. Breathe in wide into your back and ribs. As you breathe out, gently draw up the muscles of the pelvic floor as if you were stopping the flow of urine. Breathe in and gently release. These are internal muscles; make sure you are not tensing or tightening any external muscles such as the buttocks or moving out of your neutral position. There should be no visible external movement— you should feel it inside. Don't expect to feel a strong contraction—these are muscles that support you against gravity.

2 Now imagine that you are taking the pelvic floor muscles up in an elevator, one floor at a time, up to the fourth floor. What happened when you got to the top? Did the elevator crash to the bottom? Try to release down floor by floor. This control comes with time.

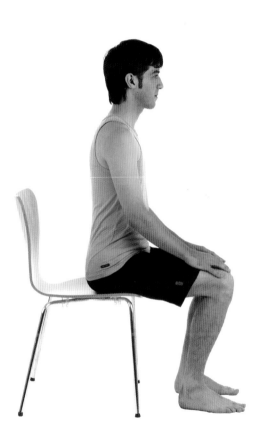

awareness

■ The pelvic floor muscles are extremely important, because they help to prevent ailments such as incontinence, prolapse, and prostate problems, and they enhance your sex life and orgasms. They are particularly important for women who have had children, as pregnancy weakens these muscles, which can lead to stress incontinence.

■ When we engage these muscles in our exercises, we draw them up to around floor two of the pelvic elevator. It is important not to grip, or create any tension—less is more in Pilates.

engaging navel to spine

It can take some time to learn how to keep the abdominals engaged on the in breath, but you will be surprised how easy it becomes if you practice Pilates regularly.

1 Get into the Relaxation Position (see page 16) and check your alignment. Place the heels of your hands on your hip bones, fingers on your pubic bone, and find a comfortable neutral position.

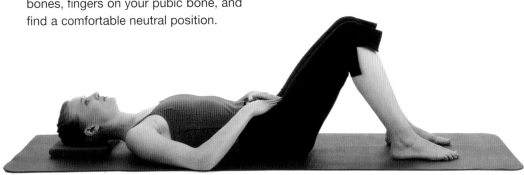

2 Breathe in wide and think of your spine lengthening. As you exhale, gently draw your navel toward your spine. Try to get the feeling of a scooping or hollowing of your abdominals. Don't grip or tense, but think of engaging these muscles with about 30% of their maximum strength.

3 This time, when you engage navel to spine, engage the pelvic floor muscles at the same time. It can be helpful to visualize smiling across your hip bones—try it and see. Imagine you have a smile drawing up from your pelvic floor muscles and spreading across to your hip bones on each side.

4 Ideally, the engagement of your abdominals should not be completely released on the in breath. See if you can keep your abdominal muscles working as you inhale. Take a wide breath in, and lengthen the spine. Exhale, and engage your abdominals and pelvic floor muscles without gripping or tensing. Now inhale, trying not to let your abdominals completely release—you can see now why you need the wide breath. As you exhale again, re-engage navel to spine, because the abdominals will have released a little with the in breath.

engaging in four point position

This is a good position for feeling the breath coming into your back, and to work the abdominal muscles against gravity.

1 Adopt the Four Point Kneeling Position (see page 25). Let your abdominal muscles relax and take a wide breath into the sides and back of your ribs.

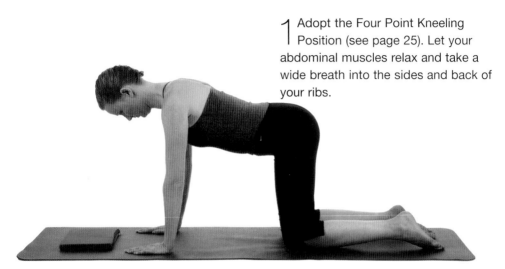

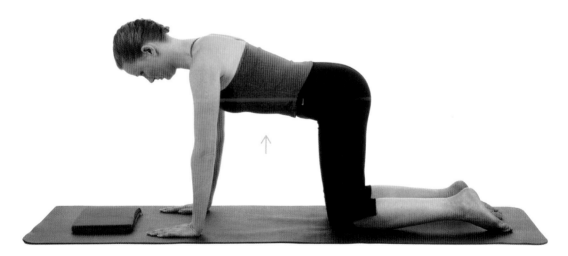

2 Exhale, draw your navel toward your spine, and engage your pelvic floor muscles. Can you see how the abdominals are lifted toward the spine, working against gravity?

3 Inhale without entirely releasing your abdominals.

4 Exhale, and re-engage your abdominals.

prone position

Here is one more common Pilates position in which you need to learn how to hold your abdominals and pelvic floors. Keep them engaged throughout this exercise, on the in breath as well as the out breath.

1 Lie on your front with your head resting on your hands. Your legs are shoulder-width apart and relaxed. Send your pubic bone to the floor. Find the neutral position for your pelvis, with hip bones and pubic bones on the same plane. You should be able to slide a $5 bill under your stomach. Inhale to lengthen the spine.

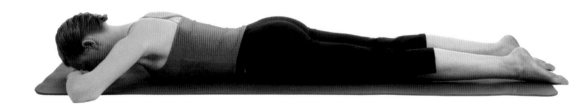

2 Exhale, drawing the pelvic floor muscles up to level 2 of the elevator and your navel toward your spine. Imagine you have a ripe strawberry under your navel and you don't want to crush it! Use your abdominal muscles to keep the pelvis in neutral.

active standing

You learned about a good standing posture on page 20. We are going to take this concept further now by using your buttock muscles in standing. Standing will never be the same again! Use Active Standing in everyday life, whenever you think of it.

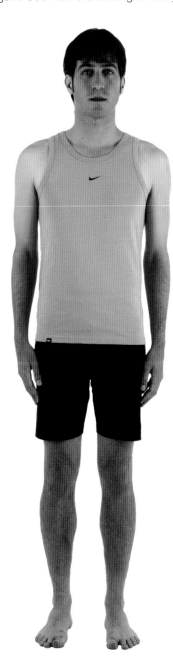

awareness

■ If you suffer from lower back pain or sciatica, sometimes the action of bringing the backs of the inner thighs together can feed into the lower back and cause tightness. If this is the case, try just thinking about the movement instead of actually squeezing. You will get some muscle activity just by thinking about the movement, and as your back releases you should be able to progress.

1 Stand with your feet hip distance apart, either parallel or slightly turned out. Check your weight is evenly distributed, and that your knees are in line with your feet and soft. Your pelvis is in neutral, your spine and neck are long. Think of the crown of your head stretching up to the ceiling as your tailbone lengthens to the floor. This doesn't mean you should tuck your tailbone under—keep it long and away, down to the floor. Now think of the back of the inner thighs coming toward each other. Imagine the muscles at the front of the inner thighs are wrapping around you to meet the muscles at the back of the inner thighs. Do your feel your pelvic floor muscles working too? Now inhale, crown of head to ceiling, tailbone to floor.

2 Exhale and draw your shoulderblades gently down your back, while bringing the backs of the inner thighs together.

active sitting

Practice Active Sitting periodically throughout the day and remember to be aware of your imaginary plumbline so that you are in good alignment.

1 Adopt the good sitting position described on page 22. Sit forward on the chair with your weight equally placed in the center of your sitting bones. There should be right angles at your hips and knees, with your knees about shoulder-width apart. Feel your feet firmly planted on the floor, helping to support your weight. Think about the plumbline running from the ear, through the front of the shoulder, and down through the hip. Imagine that the top of your head is floating upward, creating space between each vertebra, lengthening up through the spine. Visualize your tailbone dropping down, as if it is resting on the chair behind you. Now think of sitting UP instead of sitting down, with your wrap-around thigh muscles working.

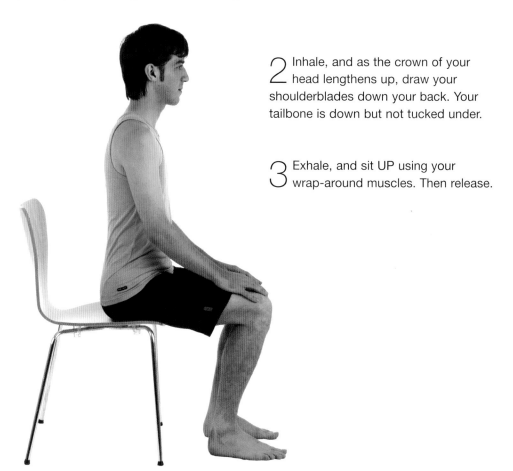

2 Inhale, and as the crown of your head lengthens up, draw your shoulderblades down your back. Your tailbone is down but not tucked under.

3 Exhale, and sit UP using your wrap-around muscles. Then release.

Keeping your knees or elbows "soft"—this means not straightening so much that you "lock" the joint.

Engaging navel to spine—this is also known as engaging your abdominals, or power house muscles. Think about hollowing or scooping these muscles.

Keep connecting—this means keeping your awareness of the muscles in question so that they are still working. It's easy to let go if you lose concentration.

Glutes—these are the hip and buttock muscles that shape your butt.

Tailbone down—this does not mean tucked under; imagine your tail on the floor behind you.

Wrap-around muscles—the action of bringing the backs of the inner thighs together, or wrapping around from the front of the inner thighs to the back, works your buttock muscles, which are important stabilizers of your pelvis.

The terms **Imagine, Visualize, Think of, Feel, See,** are used throughout the book. If you find it difficult to visualize, substitute another word that has meaning for you. For instance, you may find it easy to "imagine" your tailbone lengthening to the floor but impossible to "visualize." Likewise it may be easier for you to "think of" the crown of your head lengthening rather than "feeling" it. Experiment with different words and see what works for you.

After each exercise, you will find a section called **Awareness**. This gives additional tips for you to think about, or to bring your awareness to, in order to help you understand what you are doing.

One last thing: When you are instructed to take your awareness to a particular area or group of muscles, that means to have a sense of them working. This awareness can take some time to develop. Imagine if I were to ask you to start writing with your left foot—you wouldn't expect to be able to that for a while would you? Give yourself time—and practice.

chapter 3

warm-up

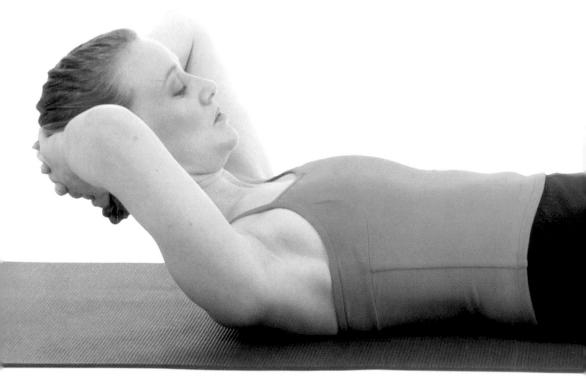

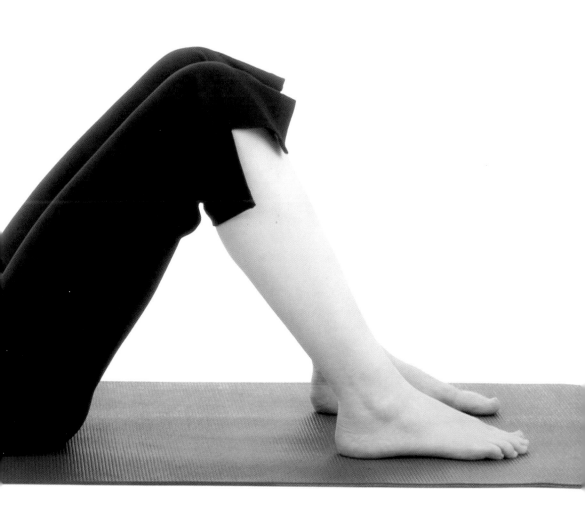

shoulder shrug

release

This exercise is good for releasing tension in the shoulders and working the muscles that draw the shoulderblades down the back. You can do it sitting at your desk at work any time your shoulders feel tight.

1 Stand in a good standing position (see page 20). Breathe in and lift your shoulders up toward your ears. As you breathe out, draw your shoulders part way down your back.

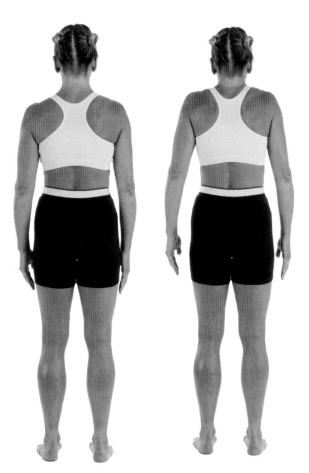

2 Breathe in and raise your shoulders up. As you breathe out, draw your shoulderblades a bit further down your back.

3 Breathe in and raise your shoulders up, then breathe out and slowly draw your shoulderblades fully down.

awareness

■ Think about the muscles around your shoulderblades that pull your shoulders down. The front of your chest and shoulders should feel wide, but avoid pushing the chest out or squeezing the shoulderblades together.

back stretch

release/stretch

To release and stretch the back and buttock muscles. This feels great if you have been standing or sitting for long periods and your back muscles are tight.

1 Lie on your back in the Relaxation Position (see page 16). Slide one heel toward your pelvis then lift your knee to your chest. Repeat with the other leg.

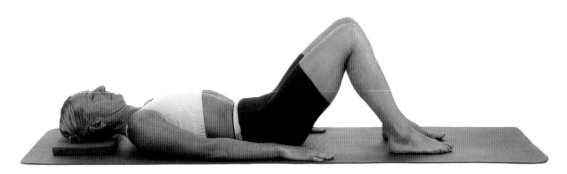

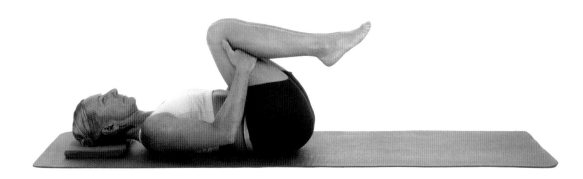

2 Hug your knees to your chest. If you have knee problems, hold under the thighs instead. Bend your elbows so that your chest and shoulders are relaxed and open. From this position, you can make tiny circles with your knees or gently rock backward and forward.

awareness

■ You'll feel a stretch in the lower back. Make sure you keep your shoulders relaxed and your chest open.

shoulder drop

release/stretch

This is another exercise, like Shoulder Shrug, where you use the back muscles to draw your shoulderblades downward. These muscles can be weak if you tend to sit hunched over a desk most of the day, and strengthening them will improve your posture.

1 Lie on your back in the Relaxation Position (see page 16). Rest your arms on the floor by your sides, with your shoulders open and relaxed. Inhale and raise the shoulders up toward your ears.

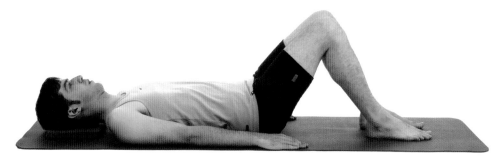

2 As you exhale, lengthen the crown of your head away as you draw your shoulderblades down your back. Stretch your fingers toward your heels. Hold this position. If you feel the muscles in your chest and the front of your shoulders working instead of the shoulderblade muscles, try imagining that your shoulders are heavy and they're sinking into the mat.

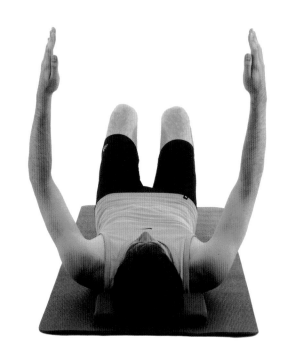

3 As you exhale, raise both arms above your shoulders, with your elbows slightly bent, palms facing each other and shoulder-width apart. Drop the back of your shoulders into the mat.

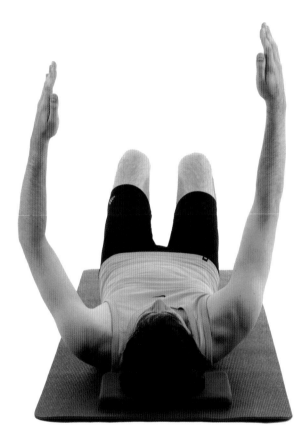

4 Breathe in and peel your right shoulderblade off the mat. Reach toward the ceiling with your right arm, stretching through the fingers.

5 Breathe out and drop your shoulder back down then draw your shoulderblades down your back. Repeat with your left arm, then do 5 more repetitions with each arm.

awareness

■ Avoid tensing the muscles in the chest or front of the shoulder. Think about keeping your chest and shoulders wide, as if you are hugging a bear!

arm opening

release/stretch

This exercise is a lovely stretch that opens up the front of the chest and shoulders. Once you can do it comfortably, try combining it with Shoulder Drop, but note that the breathing pattern is slightly different when you put the two together.

1 Lie on your back with your arms in the air, as in steps 1 to 3 of Shoulder Drop (see page 44). Breathe in and draw your shoulderblades down your back.

2 Breathe out, and move your arms in an arc down to the floor, in line with your shoulders. Keep your elbows slightly bent; don't lock them.

3 Breathe in, visualizing your collarbones widening out toward the sides of the room. Imagine you are sending your breath all the way to your fingers.

4 Breathe out and return to the starting position. Repeat 4 to 6 times.

awareness

■ As you take your arms down to the floor, imagine they are growing longer. Breathe into any areas of tension or tightness you can feel.

■ Think about the width across the front of your chest and shoulders and keep this area open.

progression—with shoulder drop

1 Lie on your back with your arms in the air, as in steps 1 to 3 of Shoulder Drop (see page 44). Breathe in and peel both shoulders off the mat at the same time. Keep your elbows slightly bent and extend your fingers toward the ceiling (a).

2 Breathe out and drop the backs of your shoulders down to the floor, then draw your shoulderblades down your back (b).

3 Breathe in and take your arms out to the floor in an arc shape, keeping them in line with your shoulders (c).

4 Breathe out and bring your arms up to the starting position, imagining the backs of your shoulders are heavy. Repeat 4 to 6 times.

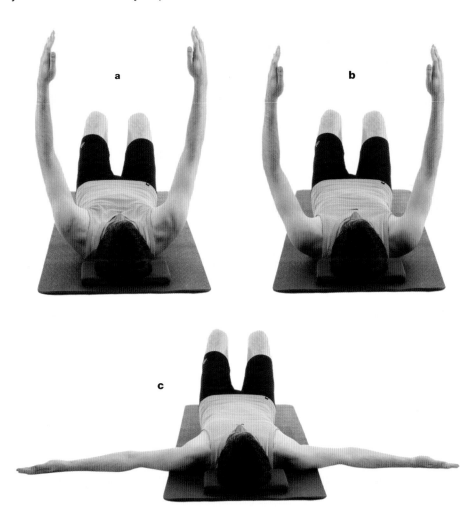

a

b

c

knee drop

stability

This is a basic stability exercise that will teach you how to keep your pelvis stable while moving your legs. It works the deep abdominal muscles, and is more difficult than it looks! When you've mastered it, try the progression with hip release movements incorporated.

1 Lie on your back in the Relaxation Position (see page 16). Take a wide breath into the sides of your ribs and lengthen your spine.

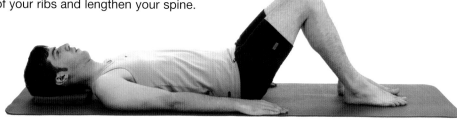

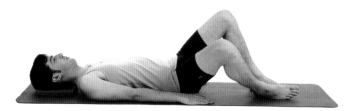

2 As you exhale, engage your abdominal muscles by drawing your navel toward your spine. Open one knee out to the side, just as far as you can without letting your pelvis move. Keep the other knee pointing toward the ceiling.

awareness

■ Keep your shoulders dropped into the floor and your hip bones level.
■ Make sure the leg that's not moving doesn't drift out to the other side to counterbalance you.
■ Think about lengthening down the front of the leg as you open it out to the side.
■ If you can feel this exercise in your lower back, try it with a flat pillow or small folded hand towel placed under your hips or lower back until your abdominals get stronger.

3 Inhale and hold this position, keeping your abdominals engaged.

4 As you breathe out, use your abdominal muscles to keep your pelvis stable as you bring your knee back to the starting position. Do 4 repetitions with each leg.

progression—with hip release

1 Follow steps 1 to 3 of Knee Drop. Exhale and slide the outside of your heel down the floor until your leg is straight. Make sure you keep your abdominals engaged and that your pelvis doesn't move (a).

2 Inhale as you turn your leg inward so that it is parallel to the other (bent) leg (b).

3 Exhale as you draw the straight leg back up to the starting position. Do 4 repetitions with each leg (c).

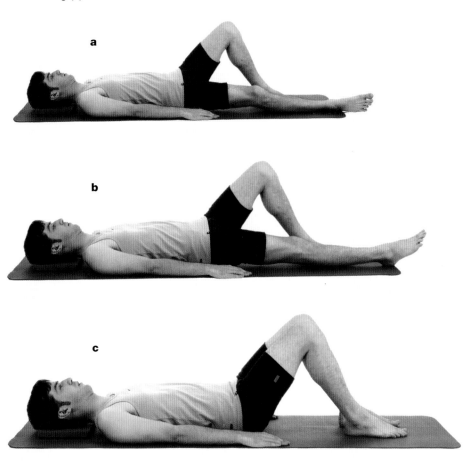

a

b

c

awareness

■ Don't let your hips roll to one side as you move your leg—keep your hips level.

spine curl

flexion of the spine/release and shoulder stability

In this exercise, you will learn how to roll your pelvis using your "power house" muscles. Spine Curl is good for easing out tight muscles in the lower back but don't try it if you have disc problems—talk to your physician to see if it is advisable in your case.

1 Lie on your back in the Relaxation Position (see page 16). Take a deep breath and lengthen your spine.

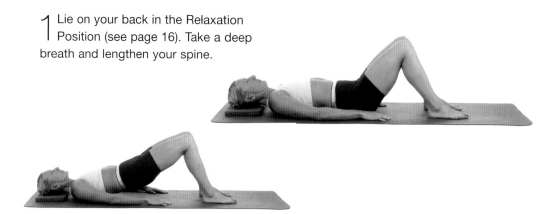

2 Breathe out and engage your abdominal muscles by drawing your navel toward your spine. Tuck your tailbone under your pelvis and you'll feel your pubic bone tilting toward your navel as your spine rolls up off the mat. Curl up until your knees, hips, and shoulders are in a straight line. (Don't worry if you can't get this far at first—just go as far as it feels comfortable.)

3 Breathe in and hold this position, keeping your abdominals engaged and your tailbone tucked under.

4 Breathe out and gradually curl back down, feeling each vertebra touch the floor. After your waist has reached the floor, slowly curl back to the starting position. Repeat 4 times.

awareness

- Think about rolling your spine upward like a wheel, rather than lifting it.
- Keep your knees in line with your hips—don't let them drift outward. Feel the length down the front of your thighs and imagine that your knees are moving toward your toes.
- Keep looking at the ceiling with the back of your neck long and shoulders down.
- If your hamstrings feel tight, press down through your heels—or stretch your hamstrings first (see page 72).

progression—with arms

1 Do steps 1 and 2 of Spine Curl. Inhale, then float your arms upward in line with your ears, just as you did in Shoulder Drop (see page 44). Keep your abdominals engaged throughout. Once you are confident doing this exercise, you can take your arms further back, but make sure the back of your ribs stay on the floor and your tailbone remains tucked under. You may need to take an extra breath (a).

2 Exhale and peel your spine down vertebra by vertebra. When you are back on the floor again, lower your arms to the starting position. Repeat 4 times (b).

a

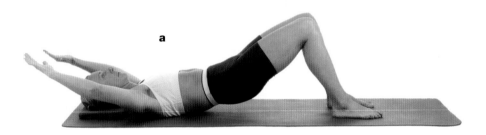

b

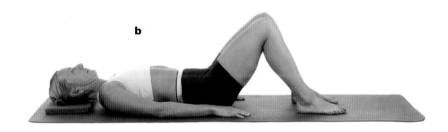

awareness

■ In the picture (right), the arms have been taken too far back. Can you see how the stability of the trunk has been lost by the ribs expanding outward?

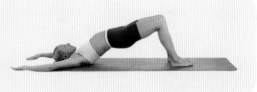

neck roll

release

You can do this with or without a pillow. It is good for releasing any tension in the neck muscles—try it either before or after you do Curl-Up.

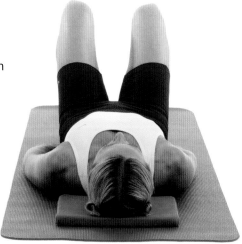

1 Lie on your back in the Relaxation Position (see page 16). Let your head sink down heavy into the floor and relax your jaw muscles by slightly opening the lower jaw.

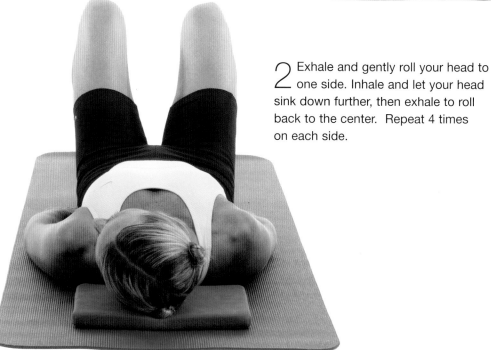

2 Exhale and gently roll your head to one side. Inhale and let your head sink down further, then exhale to roll back to the center. Repeat 4 times on each side.

head nod

release

This exercise is a way of finding the correct head and neck position, so that you don't strain your neck when curling up off the floor.

1 Lie on your back in the Relaxation Position (see page 16) Inhale and lengthen through the back of the neck, slightly dropping the chin. Don't force your chin down—keep your head on the floor.

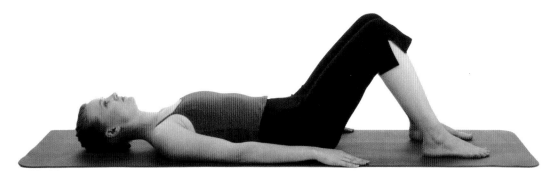

2 Lengthen through the back of the neck and slightly drop your chin. Repeat this 4 or 5 times. Always "nod" your head in this way before doing any exercise which involves lifting your upper body from the floor. Now try this with your head supported in your hands.

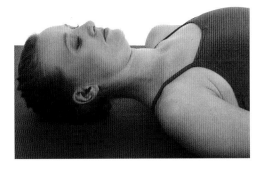

curl-up

flexion of the spine/stability of the pelvis

Curl-Up is great for giving you a flat stomach and it also teaches you how to curl your spine forward without slipping out of alignment. It will work the deep flexor muscles of the neck; if you have neck problems, do Neck Roll instead (see page 52).

1 Lie on your back in the Relaxation Position (see page 16) with your hands behind your head, supporting its weight. Inhale and gently nod your head and lengthen your spine.

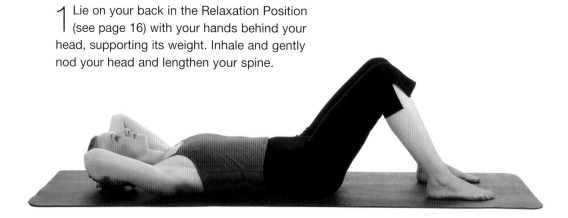

2 Exhale and engage your abdominal muscles by drawing your navel toward your spine. Curl up, lifting your head, shoulders, and upper back off the floor, looking toward your navel.

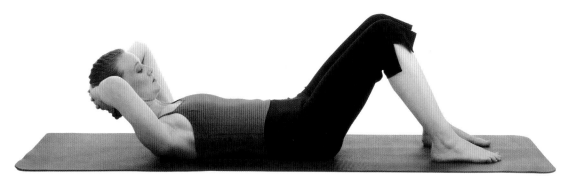

3 Keep your abdominals engaged as you inhale, then curl back down in a slow, controlled manner, as if the top of your head is lengthening away from your feet. Repeat 8 times.

awareness

- As you start to curl up, imagine you have a lead weight on your chest, dropping your breastbone down into the floor.
- Avoid pressing your lower back into the floor.
- Keep your pelvis aligned, in neutral, so that your pubic bone stays down in line with your hip bones.
- As you exhale and curl up, think about your ribs sliding down toward your pelvis.
- Feel the weight of your head in your hands, but don't pull your head up.
- This exercise uses the transverse abdominal muscles (see page 32) to give a long flat stomach. In the picture below, the deep abdominal muscles aren't engaged so the central rectus abdominus muscle (the one that gives some people a "six-pack") is causing the stomach to bulge.

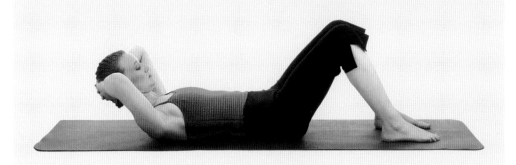

folding through

rotation/shoulder release

In this exercise you will rotate your spine while your body weight is supported on your arms and legs, which helps to build strength and bone density, especially in the wrists. It can help to prevent osteoporosis, a disease in which the bones become thin and brittle.

1 Kneel in the Four Point Position (see page 25). Breathe in and look directly down at the floor, then think about pushing down into the floor as if you are trying to push it away from you. You should feel this in your shoulderblades.

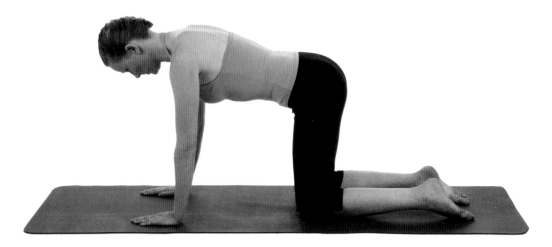

2 Breathe out and engage your abdominals by drawing your navel toward your spine. Bend your left elbow and slide your right arm underneath your chest, with the back of your right hand on the floor. Keep your spine straight right through to the top of your head.

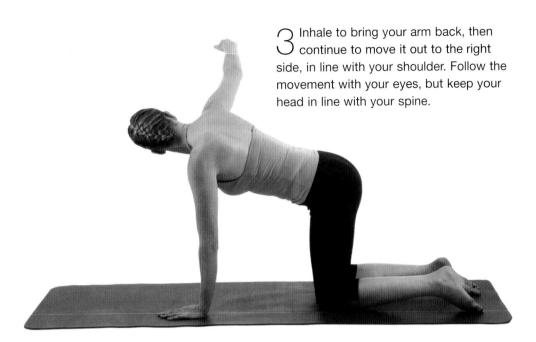

3 Inhale to bring your arm back, then continue to move it out to the right side, in line with your shoulder. Follow the movement with your eyes, but keep your head in line with your spine.

4 Exhale, keeping your abdominals engaged and pushing the floor away as you come back and repeat the movements on the other side. Do 2 repetitions on each side.

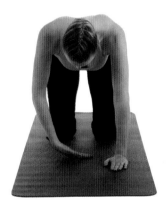

awareness

■ Spread the load from the heel of the hand all the way through to the fingers and cup your hand slightly.

■ If your wrists are uncomfortable in Four Point Position, try resting the heel of your hand on a paperback book so that the fingers are angled down slightly.

■ Keep the length between the tops of your shoulders and your ears.

■ When you take your arm out to the side, think of the movement coming from the muscles around the waist and middle of your back, not your arms.

■ Make sure your lower back doesn't arch.

upper back press

extension of the spine

This simple movement is a good way to lengthen the spine, especially if you have been doing a lot of work at a computer.

1 Lie on your front in the lying Prone Position (see page 36) with your feet and legs hip-distance apart and relaxed. Bend your elbows out to the side. Rest your forehead on your folded hands. Engage your abdominal muscles by drawing your navel toward your spine. Send your pubic bone toward the floor.

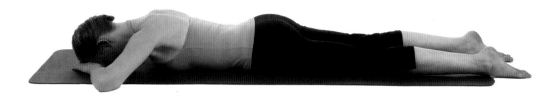

2 Breathe in, feel your spine lengthen and let your shoulders soften upward a little.

3 Breathe out, keeping your abdominals engaged. Slide your shoulderblades down your back toward your waist. Breathe in and hold.

awareness

■ Where do you feel this exercise working? Can you feel your upper back muscles working as you slide your shoulderblades down? If you feel it in your lower back, place a cushion under your stomach for the first few weeks of trying this exercise to help you to use the correct muscles.
■ Imagine there's a ripe strawberry under your navel and you don't want to squash it.

4 Breathe out and slowly release your shoulders, keeping your abdominals engaged. Repeat 6 to 8 times.

progression—head lifting

1 Repeat steps 1 to 2 of Upper Back Press. Bring your head up in line with your spine as you draw your shoulderblades down.
2 Exhale to slowly lengthen back down to the mat.

rest position

flexion of the spine

This is a lovely position to stretch out the back. It also provides a gentle stretch for the inner thighs. If you have knee problems, you may want to lie on your side in the fetal position instead—or try the Back Stretch on page 43.

1 Kneel on all fours, with your feet together and knees slightly apart. Lower your hips toward your heels. Slide your arms out in front of you to give a nice stretch down the sides of the body then bring them back to rest at your sides. Rest your forehead on the floor in front of you.

2 As you inhale, imagine sending the breath deep into the back of your ribs, then into your lower back. Exhale and let go of any tension. Take a few deep breaths like this, then return to normal breathing.

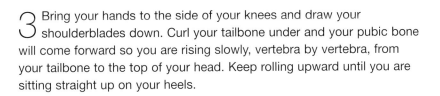

3 Bring your hands to the side of your knees and draw your shoulderblades down. Curl your tailbone under and your pubic bone will come forward so you are rising slowly, vertebra by vertebra, from your tailbone to the top of your head. Keep rolling upward until you are sitting straight up on your heels.

awareness

■ Relax your shoulders. If you can't get your forehead down to the floor, arrange some cushions so that your head and neck are supported.

chapter 4

starting off

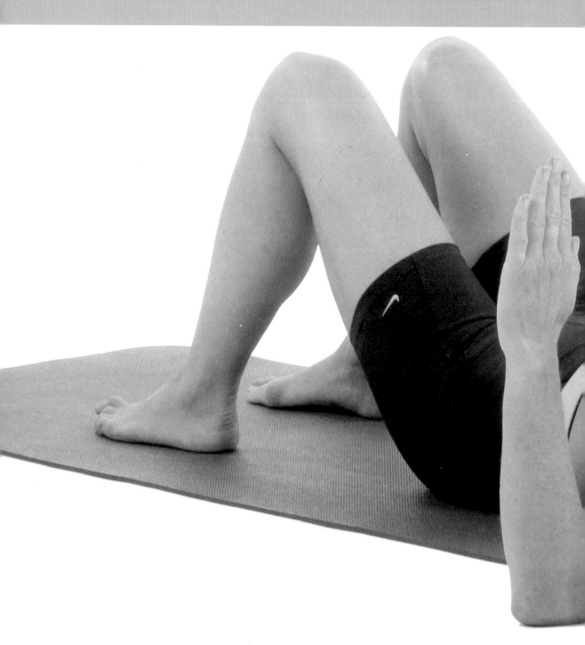

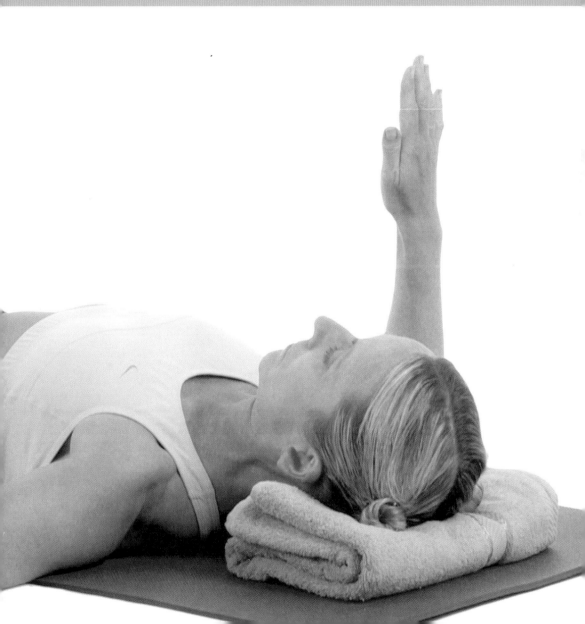

balancing

stability/extension

This exercise teaches you how to balance standing up with correct alignment. It uses the power house muscles and is a great workout for your feet, legs, and buttocks. However untrained your balance is now, with practice it will improve rapidly.

1 Stand sideways on to a chair or a wall, and place a small ball between your ankles just under your ankle bones. Maintain a good standing posture (see page 20), and rest your hand against the back of the chair or on the wall. Inhale and lengthen the crown of the head up as you draw your shoulderblades down your back.

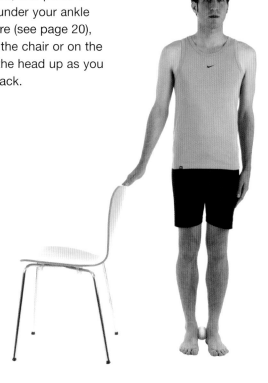

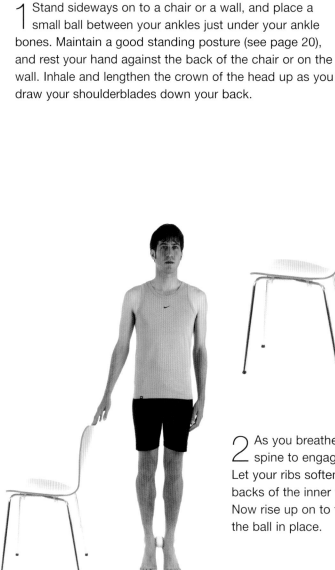

2 As you breathe out, draw your navel to your spine to engage your power house muscles. Let your ribs soften downward, and squeeze the backs of the inner thighs toward each other. Now rise up on to the balls of your feet, keeping the ball in place.

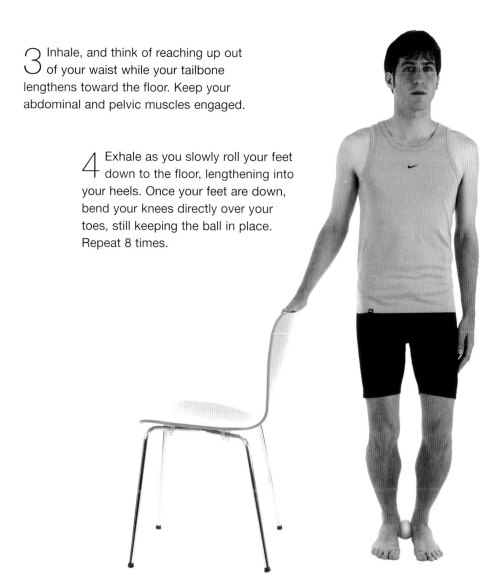

3 Inhale, and think of reaching up out of your waist while your tailbone lengthens toward the floor. Keep your abdominal and pelvic muscles engaged.

4 Exhale as you slowly roll your feet down to the floor, lengthening into your heels. Once your feet are down, bend your knees directly over your toes, still keeping the ball in place. Repeat 8 times.

awareness

■ As you rise up, imagine there are helium balloons attached to the crown of your head and try to avoid leaning forward.

■ Keep the weight evenly balanced across your toes when rising, and keep your heels down when you bend your knees.

■ When you feel comfortable with this movement, practice it free-standing. Don't worry if you wobble slightly because it means that your sensory system is having to work, which will make it sharper and better adapted to the demands of life.

floating up arms

release

This exercise teaches the correct way to move your shoulders and is good for releasing tension in the upper shoulders. There are loads of everyday movements it can help with, such as drying your hair, hanging out laundry, or lifting things off a high shelf.

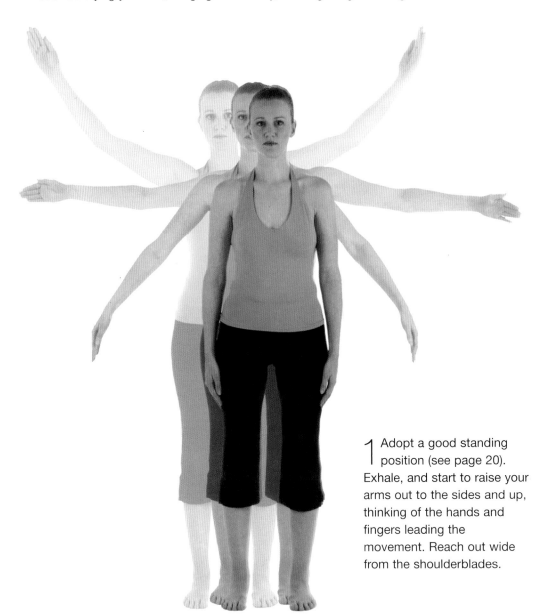

1 Adopt a good standing position (see page 20). Exhale, and start to raise your arms out to the sides and up, thinking of the hands and fingers leading the movement. Reach out wide from the shoulderblades.

2 As you are coming up to shoulder level, start to rotate your palms so that they face the ceiling. Feel your shoulderblades heavy in your back. Drop your shoulders as you raise your arms.

3 Inhale to slowly lower arms back to your sides. Repeat 4 times.

awareness

- Keep thinking about the distance between the tops of your shoulders and your ears.
- It can help to imagine you have helium balloons attached to your arms, floating them up.
- You should be releasing the upper trapezius muscles at the tops of the shoulders, and using the lower trapezius and serratus anterior muscles in the middle of the back instead. Keep saying "Drop shoulders."

variation

- This time as you exhale, float your arms forward, shoulder-width apart. Think of a ballerina gracefully bringing up her arms, reaching out and away. Keep your elbows soft, not locked. Raise to shoulder height then inhale to lower again. Repeat twice.

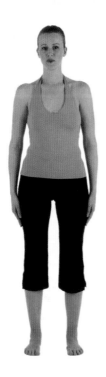
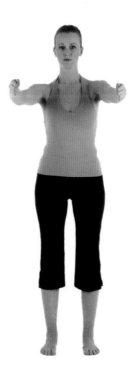

inner thigh squeeze

stability

This exercise focuses on the inner thighs and pelvic floor. It can also help to release the sacroiliac area (where the sacrum joins the bones of the pelvis), so it can be good if you suffer from sciatica, or after childbirth.

1 Lie on your back in the Relaxation Position (see page 16), but with your feet together. Place a pillow or ball between your knees. Take a wide breath into your ribs and think about your spine lengthening.

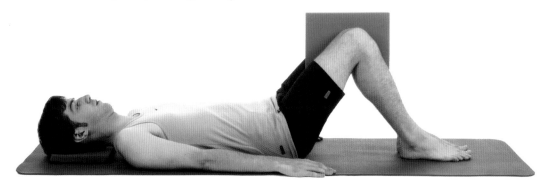

2 Exhale and engage your abdominals and pelvic floor muscles. Keeping your pelvis still, gently squeeze the pillow or ball with your knees. Think about the length down the front of your thighs.

3 Inhale, while you keep squeezing the pillow or ball. Exhale and slowly release the squeeze.

awareness

■ Keep thinking "Drop shoulders" while you do this exercise.
■ Watch that you don't grip in the front of the hips. Keep your pubic bone down—no curling.
■ Check that your lower back is not pressing into the mat, but imagine your tailbone wide and relaxed.

progression—with curl-up

1 When you are sure you can keep your pelvis in neutral, you can progress to curling up while you squeeze. Follow the instructions for step 1 opposite, but clasp your hands behind your head to support its weight. Inhale, lengthen the back of your neck, and "nod" your head (see page 53) to find its neutral position (a).

2 Exhale, engage your abdominal muscles, and draw your shoulderblades down, then curl your upper body off the mat. Keep squeezing the pillow or ball between your knees (b).

3 Inhale and look toward your navel, maintaining the distance between the tops of your shoulders and your ears.

4 Exhale, curl down to the floor again, and relax your legs.

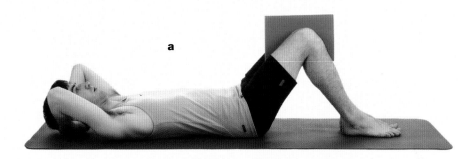

a

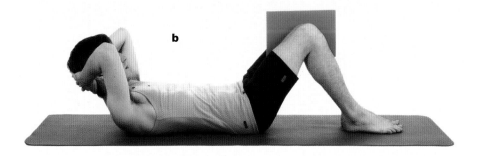

b

awareness

- Make sure your pubic bone stays down and your pelvis stays in "neutral."
- Keep those abdominal muscles and pelvic floor muscles correctly engaged.

shoulder release

release/thoracic stability

This exercise teaches you how to keep your spine stable while moving your arms. It releases the shoulders and chest and promotes mobility and flexibility. The movements are especially good for people who are round-shouldered.

1 Lie on your back in the Relaxation Position (see page 16). Reach your fingers toward your heels and then raise your arms up into the air directly above your shoulders. With your fingertips pointing to the ceiling and palms facing away from you, relax your shoulderblades into mat.

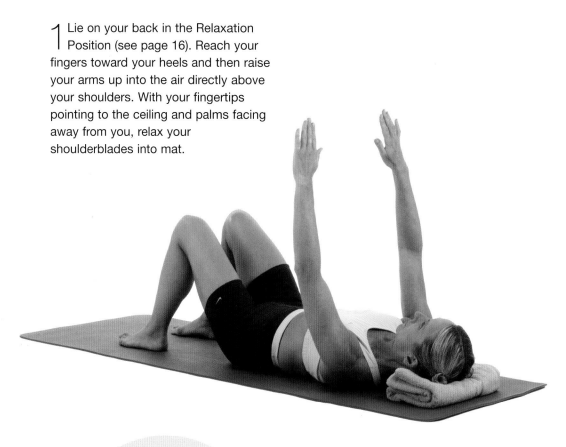

awareness

■ Did you feel your ribs or upper back moving when you took your forearms back? If so, don't take them so far—they're not meant to touch the floor.
■ Try to keep the back of your ribs on the mat. Feel your shoulderblades drawing down your back. Watch out for any tension or movement in the neck.
■ Keep the movements small enough that you can maintain alignment and control. Your range of movement will increase with practice.

2 Exhale, engage your abdominal muscles and slowly bend your elbows down to the floor, until they rest at right angles, with your arms still in line with your shoulders.

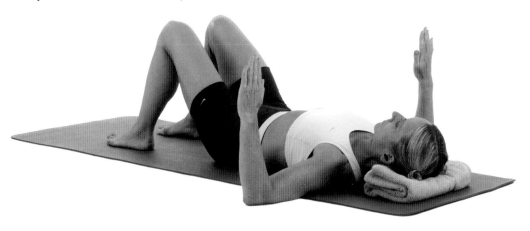

3 Inhale and take your forearms back toward the floor. Keep your ribs relaxed down and your abdominals engaged.

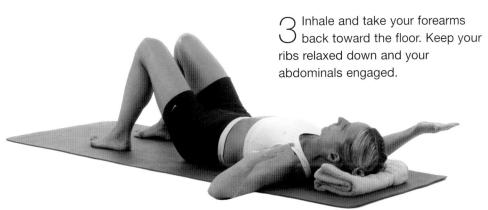

4 Exhale and reach out your arms alongside your head. Keep the back of your ribs heavy on the floor.

5 Inhale and bring your arms back to the starting position

single knee fold

stability

Here you'll learn how to keep your pelvis in neutral while moving your legs. Single Knee Fold works the deep abdominals. It is not as easy as it looks, but it's important to master this technique as a preparation for many other exercises.

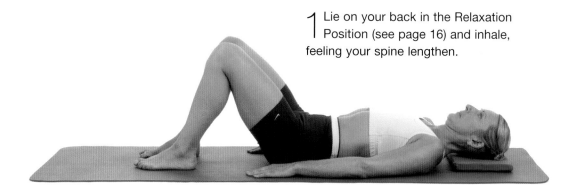

1 Lie on your back in the Relaxation Position (see page 16) and inhale, feeling your spine lengthen.

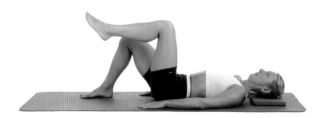

2 Exhale, engage your abdominals, and peel one foot off the floor heel first. Float the knee upward, in line with your hip. Make sure your pelvis stays in the neutral position (see page 26).

3 Inhale, and imagine the weight of your thigh bone dropping down into the floor.

4 Exhale and lower your foot to the floor—toes first, then rolling through to the heel. Repeat 4 times with each leg.

awareness

■ If you feel this in your lower back, try placing a pillow under your lower back or hips. Alternatively, move your heels closer to your hips.
■ It helps to think of the ribs coming down toward the hips as you are breathing out and engaging your abdominal muscles.
■ As you are moving your leg, say to yourself "Drop shoulders."

single leg slide

stability

This is another exercise that helps you learn how to keep a stable pelvis while moving your legs. Move slowly and focus on feeling the pelvic floor and deep abdominal muscles working, rather than the movement of the leg.

1 Lie on your back in the Relaxation Position (see page 16) and inhale, feeling your spine lengthen.

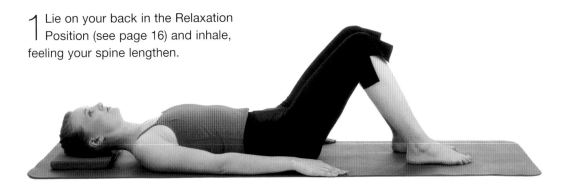

2 Exhale, engage your abdominals and soften your ribs downward. Slide one leg along the floor, keeping the other leg bent. Only lengthen the leg as far as you can while keeping a neutral pelvis (see page 26). In time, you'll be able to straighten it completely.

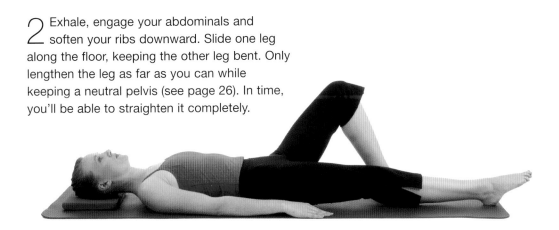

awareness

■ As you are sliding your leg, don't forget to keep your abdominals and pelvic floor muscles engaged, on the in breath as well as the out breath.

3 Inhale, as you return your leg to the starting position. You can take an extra breath and return the leg on the out breath, if you prefer. Repeat 4 times with each leg.

hamstring stretch

flexibility/release

The Hamstring Stretch will start to lengthen the hamstrings (at the backs of the thighs), which can become tight with an inactive lifestyle. You will need an elasticated scarf or band; if you don't have these, a pair of pantyhose would do.

1 Lie on your back in the Relaxation Position (see page 16) and float one knee upward. Slip the band round the sole of your raised foot. Hold the ends of the band, with your elbows bent and resting on the floor. The band should support your foot, while letting you relax the upper body, opening your chest and shoulders. Inhale and feel your spine lengthen.

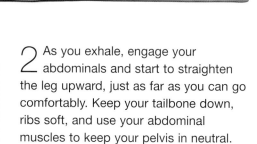

awareness

■ Remember to breathe wide into the sides and back of the ribs.
■ Keep the front of the shoulders open and down; think of your shoulderblade muscles producing the pumping action of your arms.
■ Don't allow your butt to roll off the floor, as photographed below.

2 As you exhale, engage your abdominals and start to straighten the leg upward, just as far as you can go comfortably. Keep your tailbone down, ribs soft, and use your abdominal muscles to keep your pelvis in neutral. Hold the position for about 20 seconds, breathing normally.

3 Breathe out and bend your leg then lower it to the floor again. Repeat with your other leg.

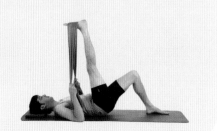

hip flexor stretch

release

The hip flexor muscles at the front of the hip get short and tight if you spend too much time sitting down, and this can lead to muscle imbalances and bad posture. The Hip Flexor Stretch will help to release and lengthen them.

1 Lie on your back in the Relaxation Position (see page 16) and inhale, feeling your spine lengthen.

2 Exhale, engage your abdominals, and float your left knee up. Hug your knee toward your chest. Inhale, and make sure that your elbows and chest are open.

awareness

■ Concentrate on keeping your upper body relaxed.
■ If you feel your lower back start to arch, don't fully straighten the leg along the floor and hug the other knee a bit closer to you.

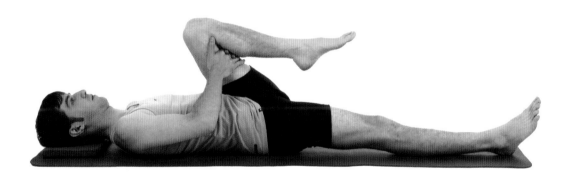

3 Exhale and slide your right leg along the floor until it is straight. Think of your ribs sliding down toward your hips so that you don't arch your lower back.

4 Inhale and think of length in your straight leg, feeling the release at the front of the hip.

5 Exhale to slide your leg back, using your abdominals to keep the pelvis stable. Repeat twice on each side.

the hundred—preparation

stability

This is a good energizer, as it improves circulation. It emphasizes lateral breathing (see page 30) and stabilization of the shoulderblades, while adding rhythm to movement. You can practice the pumping of the arms while sitting or standing as well.

1 Lie on your back in the Relaxation Position (see page 16). Inhale and, as you feel the crown of your head lengthening away, draw your shoulderblades down and point your fingers toward your heels.

2 Pump your arms up and down in small movements, close to but not touching the floor.

3 Now start to count to the following rhythm: Breathe in through the nose for 5 counts, then breathe out through the mouth for 5 counts. Keep pumping your arms as you count, and keep your abdominals engaged throughout.

awareness

■ Remember to breathe wide into the sides and back of your ribs.
■ Keep the front of the shoulders open and down; think of your shoulderblade muscles producing the pumping action of your arms.
■ You can change the count to 3 or 4, if you prefer. If you start to feel light-headed at any point, stop and rest.

four point leg slide

stability

This leg slide introduces an element of balance control and increases coordination. If it's uncomfortable for you to work on all fours, try One Leg Balance (see page 118) instead.

1 Kneel on all fours in the Four Point Kneeling Position (see page 25). Keep your neck long and look down at the floor. Breathe in and push the floor away from you.

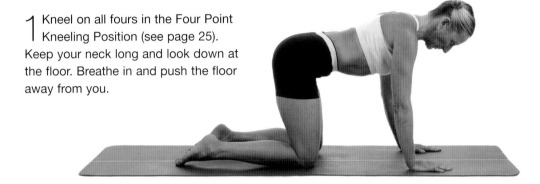

2 Exhale, engage the abdominals, and slide your right leg backward, away from you. Make sure your pelvis remains neutral and keep pushing the floor away.

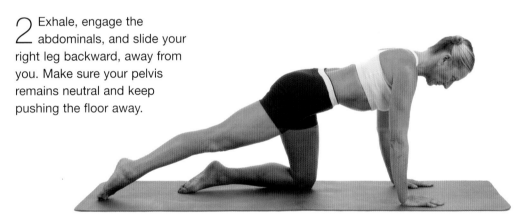

3 Breathe in and slide the leg back to the starting position. Repeat with the other leg.

awareness

■ Aim to keep both hip bones level.
■ Concentrate on balancing the weight evenly through the hands and fingers, and keeping a good distance between the shoulders and ears.

the cat

flexion

This exercise teaches you how to bend the spine, while kneeling on all fours. If you can, practice this side-on to a mirror until you have developed awareness of where your body is during the movements. If you have a disc injury, seek advice before trying The Cat.

1 Kneel in the Four Point Kneeling Position (see page 25). Press the floor away from you and check that your spine is neutral (see page 35). Breathe in wide to the back of your ribs and feel the length from the crown of your head to your tailbone.

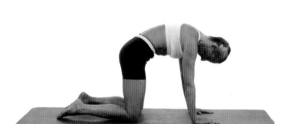

2 Exhale, engage your abdominals, and roll your tailbone under. Imagine your pubic bone curling toward your navel. Continue rounding your spine, and relax your head and neck downward. Take a wide breath in and direct it into your back.

3 Exhale, and keep engaging your abdominals as you bring your tailbone back up. This will feel as if you are slightly sticking your bottom up. Carry on bringing your spine back to the starting position, head last. Check that you are in the correct position before you do another repetition. Repeat 5 times.

awareness

■ Keep your elbows straight but make sure you don't lock them.
■ If you are rounded in the upper back (as shown below), keep your mid and upper back still and just concentrate on curling your pubic bone to navel.

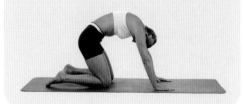

chair roll-down

release

Here, the spine is bent forward, releasing tension in the neck, shoulders, and back. This is a nice release you can do while sitting in your chair in the office. Seek advice from a physician before trying this if you have a disc injury or back problem.

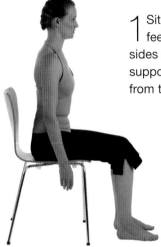

1 Sit forward in a chair, as described on page 22. Feel your feet on the floor. You can either have your arms by your sides or rest your hands on your thighs, using them to support you. Inhale to lengthen the crown of the head away from the tailbone.

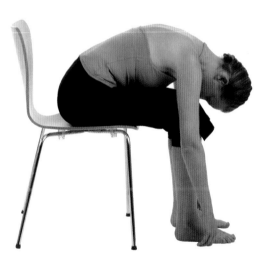

2 Exhale, engage your abdominals, and slowly let your head roll forward, as if you are peeling your spine away from a wall. Just go as far as feels comfortable.

3 Inhale, keeping your abdominals engaged. Let your neck, shoulders and arms relax.

4 Exhale and use your abdominals to roll your pubic bone toward your navel, rotating your pelvis as you slowly curl back up. Once the pelvis is in neutral position, uncurl your spine slowly, vertebra by vertebra, bringing your head back last. Repeat 4 to 6 times.

awareness

■ You may need to take an extra breath, depending on how far you manage to roll down.
■ If you are not using your arms for support, let them go loose and limp.

seated side bend

flexion

This movement, which bends the spine sideways, can be done in the office, or when you've been sitting still for long periods. The sitting position helps to isolate the movement to stop "cheating" movements in the hips.

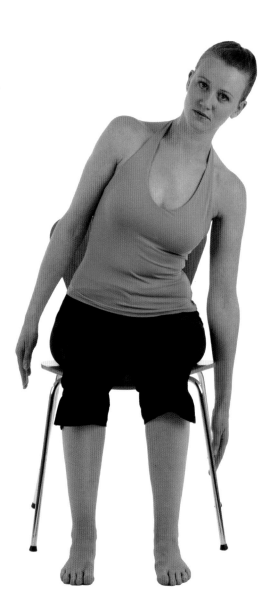

1 Sit forward in a chair, as described on page 22. Check that your pelvis is in the neutral position. Let your arms hang by your sides, with your fingers pointing down. Inhale, and lengthen the crown of the head up as the shoulders draw down.

2 Exhale, engage your abdominals, lift up out of your waist and bend to the right. Just bend as far as you can go while keeping the weight evenly balanced in your sitting bones.

3 Inhale and use your abdominal muscles to bring you back to center. Repeat 4 times on each side.

awareness

■ Drop your shoulders as you lift up out of your waist, and feel your abdominals working to stabilize the trunk. Stay long down your sides.
■ As you bend to the side, imagine you are sandwiched between two sheets of glass, so that you can't lean forward.

hip roll

This is a lovely exercise to stretch down the side of the body and to work the waist muscles—the obliques. It involves a controlled rotation of the spine.

1 Lie on your back in the Relaxation Position (see page 16), but with your feet and ankle bones together. Stretch your arms out by your sides at shoulder height (or slightly lower if you have neck or shoulder problems), with your palms facing up. Inhale, and think of length from the crown of your head to your tailbone.

2 Exhale, engage the abdominals, then drop both knees to one side as you roll your head gently to the other side. You'll feel a diagonal stretch right across your trunk. Keep the sides of your feet together, as if they are stuck with glue.

3 Inhale, and think of sending your knees away to the opposite corner of the room, to produce an extra stretch.

awareness

- Feel the length down the sides of your body as your abdominal muscles control the movement.
- You shouldn't feel this in your lower back. Don't let it arch.

4 Exhale, using your abdominals to come back to the starting position. Ribs first, then waist, pelvis, and knees last. Repeat 3 times on each side, alternating sides.

butt squeeze

extension

This exercise uses all the power house muscles of the inner thighs, buttocks, pelvic floor, and abdominals. It's a good way to learn how to keep the upper body relaxed while you are working the muscles of the lower body.

1 Lie on your front in the Prone Position (see page 36) with a small ball or cushion between your thighs. Rest your head on your hands. Point the toes of one foot toward the toes of the other, keeping your heels apart. Check that your pelvis is neutral, with your pubic bone down on the floor.

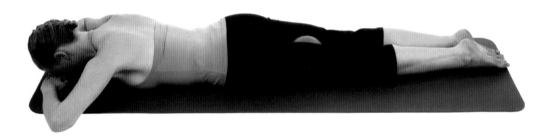

2 Exhale, drawing your navel toward your spine. Start to gently roll your heels toward each other, squeezing the ball or pillow between your thighs. Think of the back of the inner thighs coming closer to each other and the butt working.

awareness

■ If you feel this in your lower back, you may be gripping too hard with your buttocks. See if it helps to place a pillow under your stomach.
■ Keep your neck and shoulders relaxed throughout.

3 Inhale and hold this position. As you progress, you will be able to hold for longer before releasing.

4 Exhale and relax your legs back to the starting position. Repeat 6 times.

5 When you've finished, come back to Rest Position (see page 59). The Back Stretch (see page 43) is an alternative if you have knee problems, or you could roll up on your side in the fetal position.

side-lying preparation

This teaches you to find stability when lying on your side and it strengthens the muscles down the sides of the body. Take time adjusting your alignment; finding the correct position is the most important part of the exercise.

1 Lie on one side and stretch your lower arm so that you can rest your head on it and keep your spine in line. If it helps, place a small pillow between your arm and your head. If this is not comfortable, bring your arm down and let it rest in front of you in line with your shoulder, then use a thick book or firm pillow to support your head. Line yourself up so that your spine is straight: You can test this by reaching your top hand behind you and checking the distance between your spine and the edge of the mat.

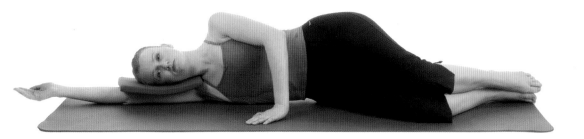

2 Bend your knees and rest your ankle bones and the sides of your feet together. Your heels should be in line with or slightly in front of your spine. Line up your trunk, so that shoulder is directly over shoulder and hip over hip. Test this with your top hand, then rest the top hand on the floor in front of you to help you balance.

3 Inhale and lengthen the crown of your head away from your sitting bones. Exhale and lengthen your sitting bones toward your heels to create length down the side of your waist. You should feel space between the floor and your waist.

4 Inhale and gently release. Repeat 3 or 4 times on each side.

the shell

stability

This is a great exercise for strengthening the sides of the butt and the hip rotators that give shape to your bottom. You will need to find a stable side-lying position, and keep your power house muscles working to maintain stability in your upper body.

1 Lie on one side and check your alignment, as described on page 81. Inhale, and send your sitting bones toward your heels to lengthen down the sides of the body.

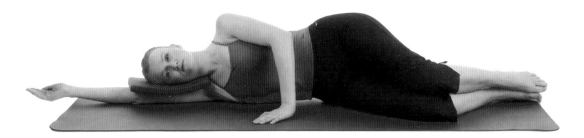

2 Exhale, engage your abdominals, and slowly lift your top knee, keeping the sides of the feet together. Focus on keeping length down the side of your body.

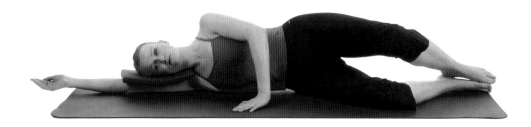

3 Inhale, draw your shoulderblades down your back, and slowly return the knee to starting position. Repeat 6 times on each side. If you are going on to the Lying Side Reach, do both exercises on one side, then turn over to repeat on the other side.

awareness

■ Keep the hip bones in line as you open the leg and don't let the hips roll back. Imagine that you have your back to a wall.

lying side reach

stability

In this exercise, you are still working on your side but the top leg is stretched out, providing an extra challenge to stability, coordination, and balance. This will strengthen the muscles of the side of the hip and leg.

1 Lie on one side and check your alignment (see page 81). Draw your shoulderblades down. Slightly bend your lower leg and straighten your upper leg in line with your body. The upper foot is stretched onto the floor, and your upper arm lies along your body with the palm face down on your thigh. Inhale, thinking of length along the sides of your body.

awareness

■ Check that you are not sinking down into your waist. Think about both sides of the waist remaining long.
■ Your eyes should look straight ahead or slightly down.

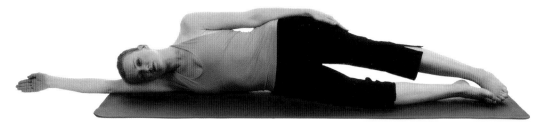

2 Exhale, engage your abdominals and lift the top leg with flexed foot until it is at hip level, simultaneously sliding your hand down your thigh. Your head will lift slightly with this movement, but don't lift it deliberately and make sure it stays in line with your spine.

3 Inhale and lower your leg and head. Repeat 6 to 8 times on each side.

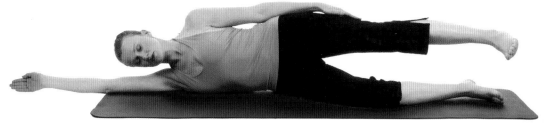

moving on

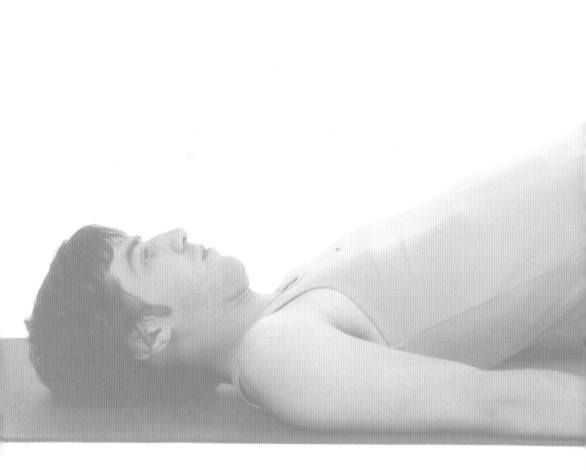

- spine curl with heel lift
- the hundred—with abdominals
- single leg preparation
- oblique curl-up
- roll back with band
- seated rotation

- opposite arm and leg lift
- press-up
- butt squeeze with press
- arm circle

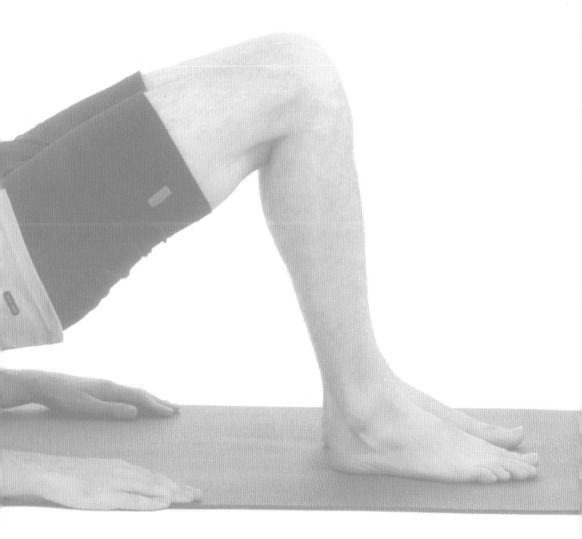

standing roll-down

flexion   chair roll-down (see page 77) is a preparation for this exercise

This exercise eases out tension in the back, neck, and shoulders, and mobilizes the spine. It increases awareness of correct abdominal stabilization when you're bending forward. If you have a back problem, seek the advice of your physician before trying it.

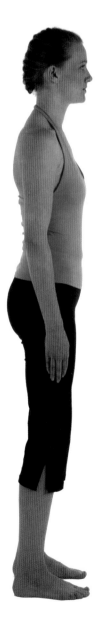

awareness

■ You may need to take an extra breath depending on how far you go.
■ Place your hands on your thighs for support if necessary.
■ Keep your abdominals engaged toward your spine throughout.
■ If your knees come toward each other as you are rolling up or down, gently squeeze the backs of your inner thighs together (see page 37).
■ Keep your body weight centered.

1 Stand with good posture (see page 20) with your knees slightly bent and eyes looking straight ahead. Inhale to lengthen your spine through the crown of your head, gently drawing your shoulderblades down your back.

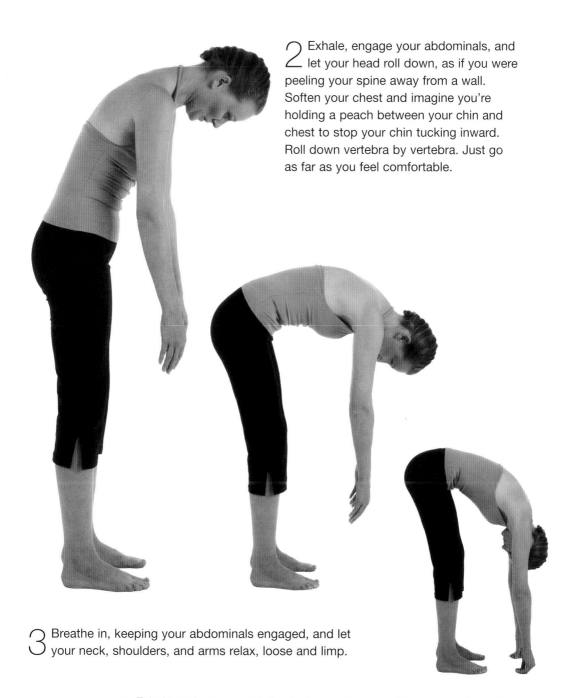

2 Exhale, engage your abdominals, and let your head roll down, as if you were peeling your spine away from a wall. Soften your chest and imagine you're holding a peach between your chin and chest to stop your chin tucking inward. Roll down vertebra by vertebra. Just go as far as you feel comfortable.

3 Breathe in, keeping your abdominals engaged, and let your neck, shoulders, and arms relax, loose and limp.

4 Exhale and use your abdominals to roll your pubic bone up toward your navel, rotating your pelvis under as you slowly reverse the roll-down. Once the pelvis is in neutral, roll up again, vertebra by vertebra, bringing your head back last. Repeat 4 to 6 times.

shoulder roll

release

You can do this simple movement to release shoulder and neck tension any time, anywhere. It's especially beneficial if you spend a lot of time sitting at the computer.

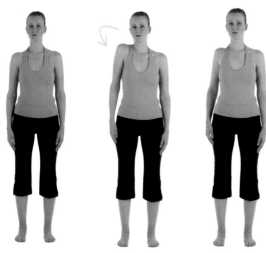

1 Stand in a good standing posture (see page 20) and think of drawing a circle with the tip of one shoulder. Take it forward, up, back, and round. As you do this, imagine the crown of your head floating up to the ceiling and keep your tailbone down.

2 Repeat 4 times with each shoulder, alternating sides.

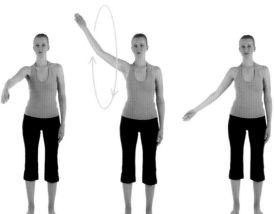

3 Now make the movement with the whole shoulder, so that you are circling the arm. Start with small circles, and gradually make them larger but stay within a comfortable range of movement. Keep your elbows slightly bent or soft. Repeat 4 times on each side.

awareness

■ Your hips might have a tendency to turn as your shoulder movements get bigger. Imagine you have headlights on your hip bones which are shining on the wall in front of you, and aim to keep them shining straight forward.

arm opening

stability/extension

This movement opens out the front of the chest and shoulders, while helping you to become aware of the stabilizing muscles of the shoulderblades. It's good if you have had shoulder injuries, as it strengthens the weaker rotator muscles of the shoulder joint.

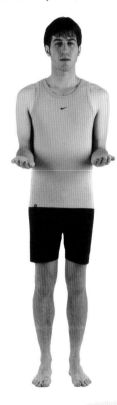

1 Stand in a good standing position (see page 20), with your bent elbows "glued" to your sides and your palms facing upward. Inhale to lengthen the crown of the head up as the shoulderblades draw down the back.

2 Exhale, keeping the shoulderblades down the back and lengthen through the fingers. Engage your abdominals.

3 Inhale as you open your forearms to the sides, leading with your thumbs. Your elbows should stay "glued" to your sides, and you should feel the muscles of your shoulderblades doing the work.

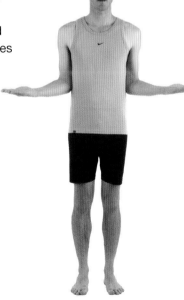

awareness

■ Stay neutral throughout (see page 24). There can be a tendency to arch the back as you open the arms, so keep engaging the abdominals.
■ Don't try to open your arms too wide.
■ Run through the following checklist: Tailbone long, navel toward spine, elbows by your sides, shoulderblades down your back, neck long.

4 Exhale to return your arms to the starting position. Repeat 6 times.

balance and float arms

stability   balancing (see page 62) is a preparation for this exercise

In Starting Off you learned to balance, but this time you will be bringing up your arms at the same time. This may make you feel more wobbly, but the adjustments your muscles make to retain balance will sharpen your balance reflexes for everyday life.

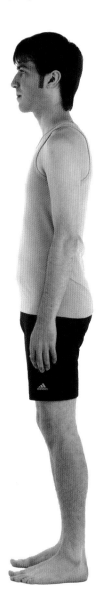

awareness

■ As you rise up, think of helium balloons attached to the crown of your head floating you up, and try to avoid leaning forward.
■ Keep the weight evenly balanced across all your toes when rising, and keep your heels down when you bend your knees.
■ As you float up your arms, think of a ballet dancer gracefully reaching out and away, with soft elbows.
■ Maintain the length between the tops of your shoulders and ears.

1 Stand in a good standing posture (see page 20). Inhale to lengthen your spine through the crown of your head, gently drawing your shoulderblades down your back.

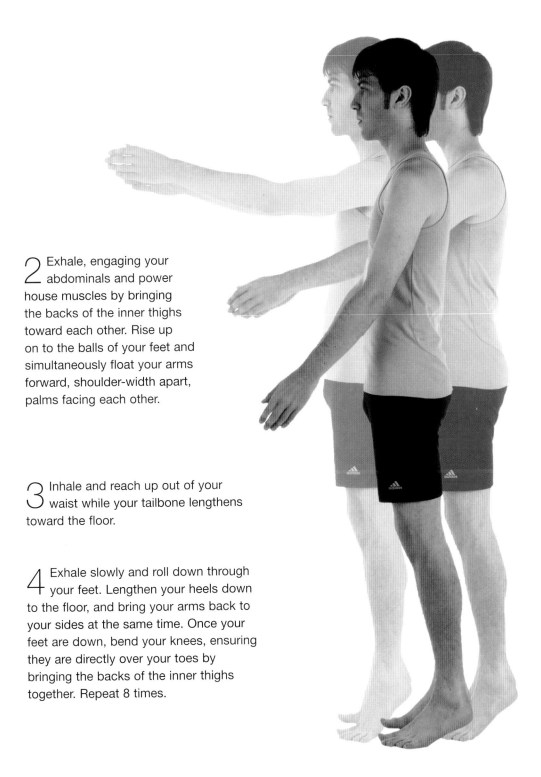

2 Exhale, engaging your abdominals and power house muscles by bringing the backs of the inner thighs toward each other. Rise up on to the balls of your feet and simultaneously float your arms forward, shoulder-width apart, palms facing each other.

3 Inhale and reach up out of your waist while your tailbone lengthens toward the floor.

4 Exhale slowly and roll down through your feet. Lengthen your heels down to the floor, and bring your arms back to your sides at the same time. Once your feet are down, bend your knees, ensuring they are directly over your toes by bringing the backs of the inner thighs together. Repeat 8 times.

standing side bend

flexion   seated side bend (see page 78) is a preparation for this exercise

Now you're ready to bend the spine sideways while standing. This improves flexibility and mobility, and gives a lovely stretch down the sides of the body. Start with your arms by your sides first and practice in front of a mirror before you progress to the long arm version.

1 Stand with good posture (see page 20) and bend your knees a little. Your arms should be down by your sides, with your fingers together and pointing down. Inhale, and lengthen the crown of the head up as the shoulderblades draw down.

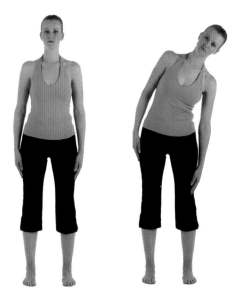

awareness

- Focus on balancing your weight evenly between both feet.
- As you bend to the side, imagine you are sandwiched between two sheets of glass, so you can't lean forward.
- Don't let your shoulders come up or your hips move to one side, and avoid bending one knee more than the other, as in the photograph below.

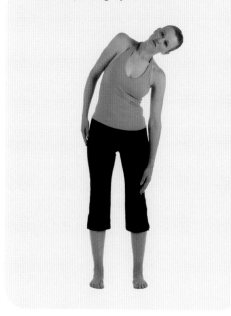

2 Exhale, engage your abdominals and lift up out of your waist then bend sideways to the right. Think of the left hip drawing away from the left rib, creating length.

3 Inhale and use your abdominals to bring you back to center, keeping your side muscles long. Repeat 4 times on each side.

progression—with long arms

1 Stand in a good posture, with your knees slightly bent. Reach your right arm straight up alongside the right side of your head. Drop your shoulder.

2 Inhale and imagine you are lifting up out of your waist and reaching the fingers of your right hand to the ceiling. You can let your shoulder go now, to get a nice stretch down the side of the body (a).

3 Exhale and engage your abdominals. Slightly bend your right elbow and reach across the top of your head. Imagine someone gently pulling your arm over and away to the opposite corner of the ceiling (b).

4 Inhale, holding this position, and breathe wide into your ribs.

5 Exhale and use your abdominals to bring you up but keeping the length down your sides. Repeat twice on each side, alternating sides.

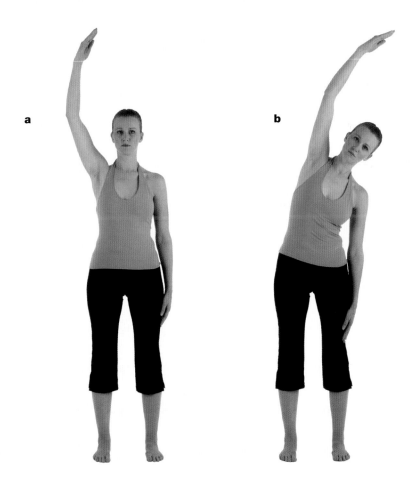

a

b

double knee fold

stability   single knee fold (see page 70) is a preparation for this exercise

You're aiming to keep the pelvis in neutral, while bringing up one knee then the other. The Double Knee Fold is the starting position for a number of exercises, and is a challenging movement in itself, as you have to keep your pelvis absolutely still throughout.

1 Lie on your back in the Relaxation Position (see page 16) and inhale to lengthen your spine.

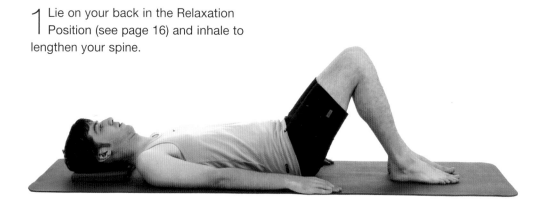

2 Exhale, engage your abdominals, and feel the heaviness of your shoulders and tailbone on the floor. Peel the right foot off the floor heel first, and float your right knee up so that your knee is at right angles to your hip. Your shin should be parallel to the floor and your foot softly pointed. Make sure your tailbone stays down and your pelvis is neutral.

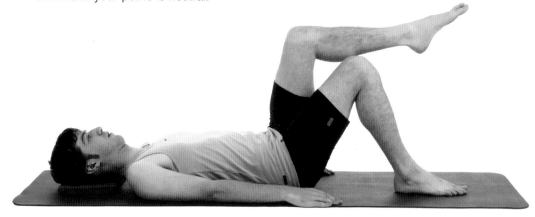

3 Inhale, and think about the hip bone dropping down into the floor.

4 Exhale, keeping your abdominals engaged and shoulderblades down. Peel your left heel up and float your left knee upward until it is at right angles to your hip and your left shin is parallel to the floor.

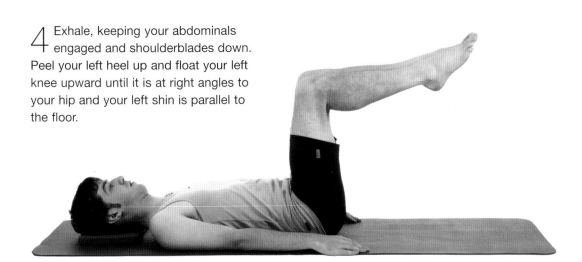

5 Inhale, keep engaging your abdominals, and start to take the left leg down again, toes first. When you reach the floor, roll through your foot from toes to heels.

6 Exhale and bring the right foot down in the same way. For the next repetition, start with the left leg first. Repeat 4 times on each side.

awareness

■ If you feel this working in your lower back, try starting with your heels closer to your hips, or place a pillow under your lower back.
■ It helps to think of your ribs moving closer to your hips and your lower back softening down into the floor, as you are moving the legs.
■ Could you keep your shoulders down or were they trying to help out? As you are moving your leg, keep reminding yourself to drop your shoulders.

spine curl with heel lift

stability/flexion   spine curl (see page 50) is a preparation for this exercise

This exercise takes the basic Spine Curl a stage further. It will challenge your power house muscles and stabilization, and you'll feel your butt muscles working hard.

1 Lie on your back in the Relaxation
Position (see page 16), thinking about the
contact between your feet and the floor. Take
a wide breath in to your ribs, to lengthen and
prepare for movement.

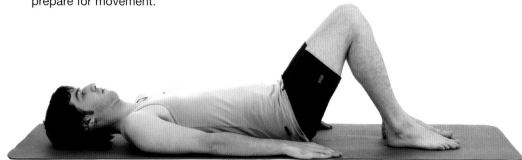

awareness

■ Think of rolling, not lifting, as you peel your spine up like a wheel. Imagine you are growing 2 inches between each vertebra.
■ The top of the movement should be no higher than knees, hips, and shoulders in line.
■ Keep your tailbone tucked under and your pubic bone toward your chin.
■ Don't let your shoulders work to stabilize you—keep them dropped down and open.
■ As you peel up the right heel you should feel the glutes on the left side working to help keep your pelvis level. Think about these muscles as you squeeze the backs of the inner thighs toward each other.
■ Try placing your hands on your hip bones to make sure they don't move when you lift your heel.

2 Exhale, engage your abdominals, drop your shoulders, and slowly curl
your tailbone under. You'll feel your lower back having more contact with
the floor. Keep peeling up your spine, vertebra by vertebra, until your knees,
hips, and shoulders are in a straight line—or lower, if it doesn't feel
comfortable to go this far.

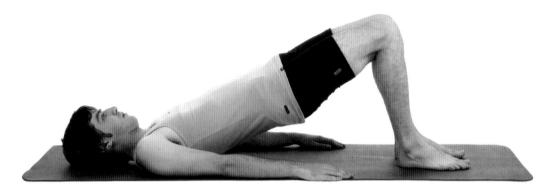

3 Inhale, and focus on keeping your hip bones level.
Remember to keep your abdominals engaged and
your ribs softened downward.

4 Exhale and focus on your strong
center as you peel the right heel up
off the floor, keeping the toes down. Make
sure nothing else moves!

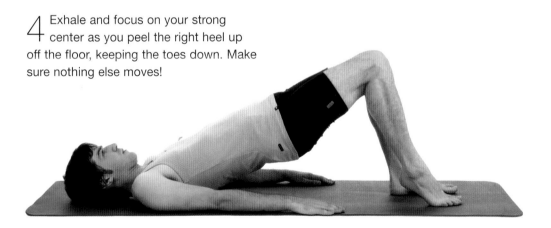

5 Inhale and roll the heel down again.
Repeat with the left heel. (If you want
more of a challenge, try doing 4 heel lifts
on each side at the top of your Spine
Curl. This is hard work!)

6 Exhale, soften your ribs downward
and wheel your spine down the floor
again, vertebra by vertebra. Repeat the
sequence 6 times.

the hundred—with abdominals

stability/flexion   the hundred (see page 74) is a preparation for this exercise

You should have mastered coordinating the breathing and arm movements from the Starting Off version of The Hundred before you try this. In Intermediate, we will challenge the abdominal muscles more.

1 Lie on your back in the Relaxation Position (see page 16) and bring your knees up, as in Double Knee Fold (see page 94). Rest your arms on the floor by your sides.

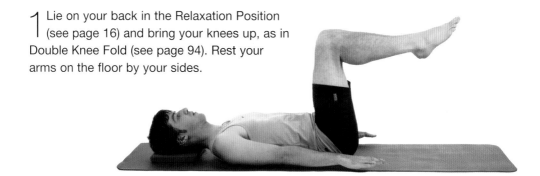

awareness

■ Think of the muscles of your upper back moving your arms. Keep the front of the shoulders open and down.
■ If you feel your lower back working, bring your knees closer toward you. As you get stronger, aim to hold them in line with your hips. Your lower back should be in contact with the floor, tailbone down.
■ You can change the count to 3 or 4 if you prefer, remembering to breathe wide into the sides and back of your ribs. Stop if you feel light-headed.

2 Inhale and reach your fingers toward your heels, drawing your shoulder-blades down your back. Pump your arms up and down in a small movement, close to but not touching the floor.

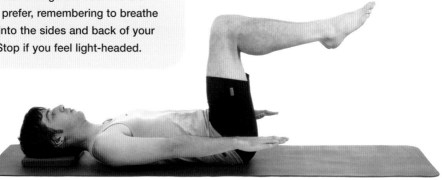

progression—with curl-up

With the upper body lifted, the deep neck flexors are working with the abdominals. This is an excellent exercise for abdominal strength and trunk stability. If your neck gets tired, rest your head on a pillow.

1 Follow the instructions for step 1 of The Hundred, opposite. Inhale and nod your head to find the correct neck position (see page 53).

2 Exhale, engage your abdominals, and curl your upper body off the floor, looking toward your navel. Try to feel your chest and back sinking into the floor as you engage navel to spine.

3 Breathe in through your nose to a count of 5 and out through your mouth to a count of 5, pumping your arms up and down. If you feel any strain or discomfort in your neck, support your head with one arm and pump with the other, then change arms halfway through. Repeat 20 times. If you can't do the full 100, start with 20 or 30 and gradually increase until you can complete without neck tension.

4 Inhale and lower your head to the floor, then bring down your legs, one at a time, in a controlled manner.

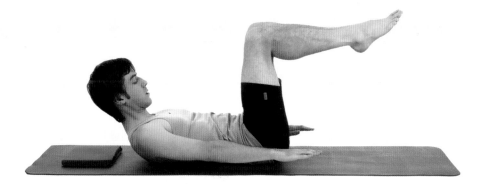

3 Now start to count to the following rhythm: Breathe in through your nose to a count of 5; Breathe out through your mouth to a count of 5. Keep pumping your arms in rhythm with your breath for 100 beats.

4 Lower your knees one by one to the starting position.

single leg preparation

stability

This will prepare you for the coordination and abdominal strength that you will need in the Single Leg Stretch (see page 126), where both legs will be lifted off the floor. It strengthens the abdominal core muscles and improves flexibility in the hip flexors and hamstrings.

1 Lie on your back in the Relaxation
Position (see page 16). Exhale, engage
your abdominals, and peel your right foot
off the floor, heel first. Float your right
knee up so that it is at right angles to
your hip with your shin parallel to the floor
and your foot softly pointed.

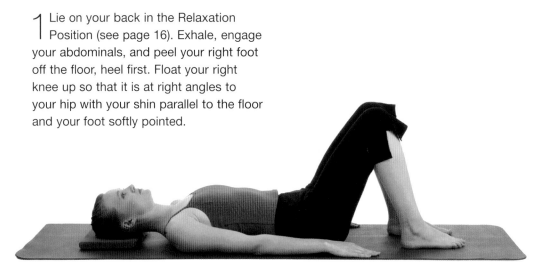

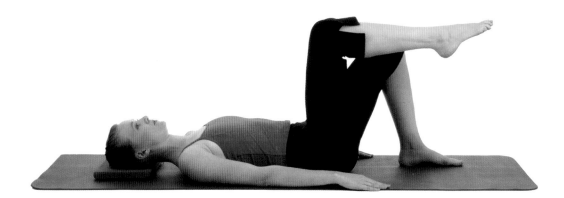

2 Inhale, and focus on the length between the crown of your head and your tailbone.

3 Exhale, re-engage your abdominals, and lengthen your right leg away from you, keeping your right knee level with the left. Let your ribs drop down and keep your spine in neutral (see page 26).

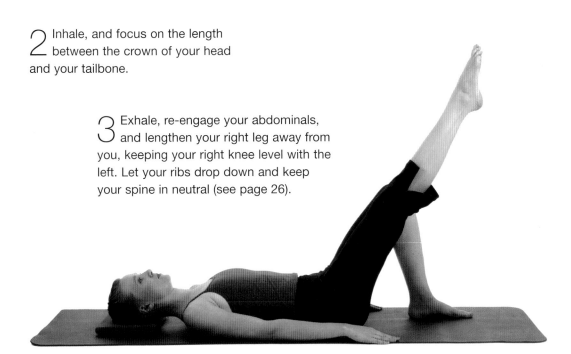

4 Inhale and return your right leg to the starting position. Repeat 4 times, then change legs and do 4 repetitions with your left leg.

awareness

■ As in the other stabilization exercises where you are lengthening an arm or a leg, the pelvis can roll and pull the spine out of neutral. If you feel lower back discomfort, this may be what is happening. Try placing a flat pillow under your lower back or hips, or don't fully straighten the working leg.

oblique curl-up

flexion   curl-up (see page 54) is a preparation for this exercise

This will strengthen the oblique muscles that wrap around the sides of your abdomen. If you have neck problems, it would be best to avoid this exercise and do Knee Drop (see page 48) or Single Leg Slide (see page 71) instead.

1 Lie on your back in the Relaxation Position (see page 16) with your hands clasped behind your head, supporting it. Check your alignment and make sure your pelvis is neutral. Inhale to gently nod your head (see page 53) and lengthen your spine.

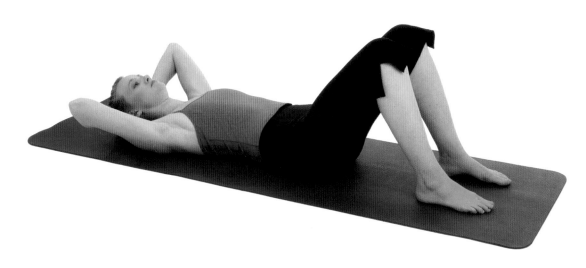

2 Exhale, engage your abdominals, and think of relaxing the area round your breastbone. Curl your upper body up and to the right, so that your left ribs draw closer to your right hip bone. Look toward the outside of your right thigh. Keep your pelvis neutral.

3 Keep the abdominals engaged as you inhale and slowly curl back down. Repeat 4 times on each side.

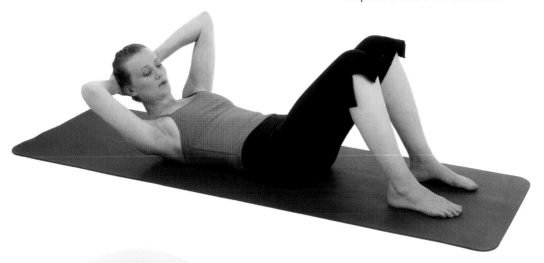

awareness

■ As you curl up, try to feel as if there is a weight on your chest making it heavy. Think of your ribs sliding down toward your pelvis. Don't roll to the side, as in the photograph below.

■ Feel your head heavy in your hands, but don't pull on it—let your abdominals do the work.

■ Maintain the distance between your shoulders and ears.

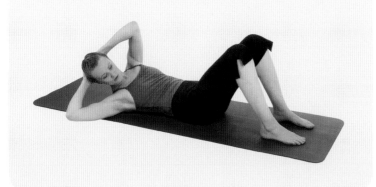

roll back with band

flexion spine curl (see page 50) is a preparation for this exercise

This is a fantastic exercise for increasing the flexibility of your lower back and learning how to control your spine, segment by segment. It uses all your power house muscles. You will need a stretch band and a folded towel or thin pillow.

1 Sit on the floor in a good sitting position (see page 23) and place a small pillow between your knees. Loop the band around the middle of the soles of your feet. Hold the ends of the band so that your arms are straight, with your shoulderblades drawn down your back. Your hands will be in the mid-calf or ankle area, depending on your build. Inhale to lengthen the crown of your head away from your tailbone.

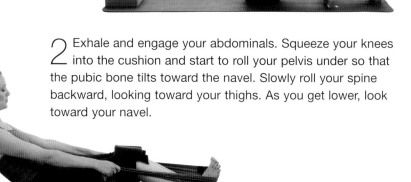

2 Exhale and engage your abdominals. Squeeze your knees into the cushion and start to roll your pelvis under so that the pubic bone tilts toward the navel. Slowly roll your spine backward, looking toward your thighs. As you get lower, look toward your navel.

awareness

- This is a complex movement. It helps to try it side on to a mirror so you can check that you are rolling down like a wheel.
- The first movement is of your pelvis rolling under. Imagine your spine in a C shape as you roll back. Don't try to lean back with a straight spine.
- Keep the front of your shoulders and your chest open and shoulderblades down.
- Your feet should stay down on the floor; move them closer to you if it helps.

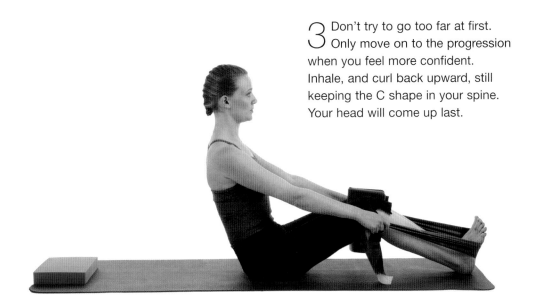

3 Don't try to go too far at first. Only move on to the progression when you feel more confident. Inhale, and curl back upward, still keeping the C shape in your spine. Your head will come up last.

progression—curling down to the floor

1 As you increase in flexibility and strength you will be able to curl down right to the floor. Position a pillow for your head to rest on and keep your head in line with your spine as you curl down. Follow steps 1 and 2 opposite and, as you take yourself back to the floor, keep looking toward your navel so that your chin doesn't point up. You may find you need to take an extra breath (a).

2 Inhale and nod your head ready to curl up. Exhale and think of lengthening your spine as you start to curl up, vertebra by vertebra. Use the band to help you keep the C shape in your spine. Keep your shoulderblades drawn firmly down your back, pelvis down, and tailbone tucked under for as long as you can.

a

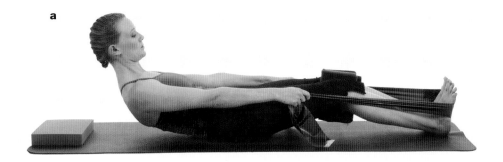

seated rotation

rotation of the spine   neutral sitting position (see page 23) is a preparation for this exercise

We all have to rotate our spines in daily life, but the rotational flexibility can easily be lost if it is not practiced. This exercise is especially useful if you have trouble kneeling and can't manage Folding Through (see page 56). You can do it sitting in a chair, if you prefer.

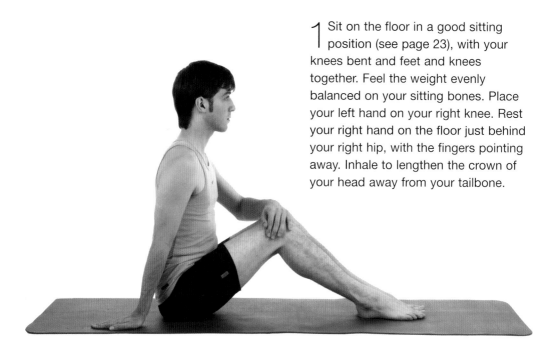

1 Sit on the floor in a good sitting position (see page 23), with your knees bent and feet and knees together. Feel the weight evenly balanced on your sitting bones. Place your left hand on your right knee. Rest your right hand on the floor just behind your right hip, with the fingers pointing away. Inhale to lengthen the crown of your head away from your tailbone.

awareness

■ It's easy to rotate the neck instead of the mid back in this exercise; to avoid this, focus your eyes on an object before you move, then as you rotate imagine your eyes tracking slowly round, with your head staying in line with the spine.
■ Focus on keeping your weight evenly balanced on both sitting bones—if you feel a slight rolling or weight shift, don't rotate as far.
■ Visualize the front of the chest and shoulders wide. There can be a tendency for the shoulder to rise up toward the ear on the side you are turning toward, but avoid this by keeping your shoulderblades drawn down your back.
■ If you need to, bend your rear elbow to maintain the distance between the top of the shoulder and your ear.

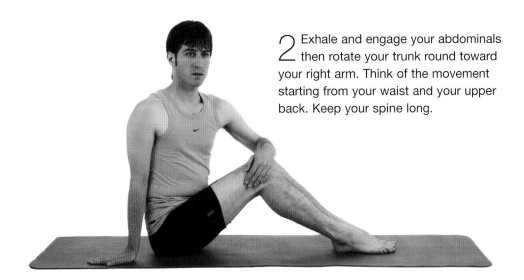

2 Exhale and engage your abdominals then rotate your trunk round toward your right arm. Think of the movement starting from your waist and your upper back. Keep your spine long.

3 Inhale, breathe into your upper back and ribs and feel the expansion there. See if you can rotate a little bit further.

4 Exhale to return to the starting position, then rotate to the left. Repeat 4 times in each direction.

progression—with straight legs

You will need to have a good length in your hamstring muscles to do this version.

1 Sit on the floor and make sure your pelvis is neutral. Straighten your left leg in front of you and bend your right leg. Your right foot can be either on the inside or the outside of the left knee. Inhale to lengthen. As in step 1 opposite, place your left hand on your right knee and your right hand on the floor behind you.
2 Exhale, engage your abdominals and rotate round to the right from the waist and upper back. Keep your weight evenly distributed on your sitting bones.
3 Inhale and pull the right knee gently toward you with your left hand. Exhale to return.

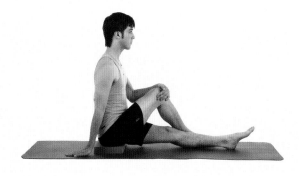

opposite arm and leg lift

four point leg slide (see page 75) is preparation for this exercise

This movement will test your balance and coordination. It works the deep abdominals, the obliques that wrap round the sides of your waist, the shoulderblade stabilizers, and the glutes (or buttock muscles).

1 Kneel in the Four Point Kneeling Position (see page 25), looking down at the floor between your hands. Inhale, press the floor away and feel the shoulder stabilizer muscles working. Keep length between the tops of the shoulders and the ears.

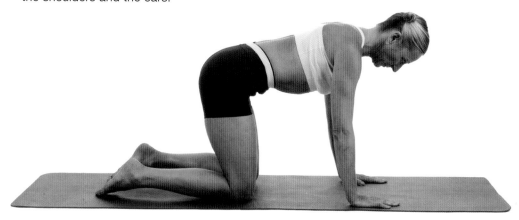

2 Exhale, engage your abdominals, and lift your left leg out and back at hip height, simultaneously floating your right arm straight out at shoulder height. Keep your shoulderblades down and your pelvis level.

3 Inhale and lower your arm and leg in a smooth, controlled manner. Repeat with the right leg and left arm. Do 4 repetitions on each diagonal.

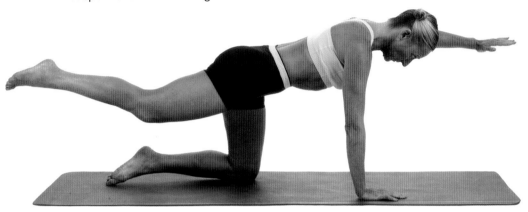

awareness

■ Visualize the arm and the leg lengthening away from your center in parallel, as if the leg is trying to reach the wall behind you and the arm the wall in front.
■ The real challenge is not losing the distance between shoulder and ear.
■ Think of the hip bones facing directly down toward the floor—don't let the weight sink into one side. In the photograph below, the weight has shifted to the right and the shoulder has come up to the ear.
■ Make sure the raised leg is in line with your hip but no higher.
■ Keep looking down at the floor with a long neck, and focus on keeping in neutral so that your lower back doesn't dip downward.

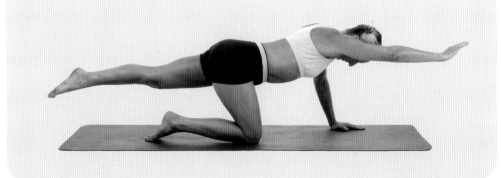

press-up

stability

Press-Up strengthens the chest, shoulders, and upper back muscles, while the abdominal muscles are stabilizing your trunk and keeping you in neutral throughout the movement.

1 Kneel on all fours with your hands slightly wider than shoulder-width apart. Your fingers face forward, and the weight is evenly distributed from the heels of the hands to the fingers. Make sure your knees are in line with your hips. Check that you are in neutral and looking down at the floor between your hands. Inhale and think of lengthening between the crown of the head and the tailbone. Press the floor away to draw your shoulderblades down.

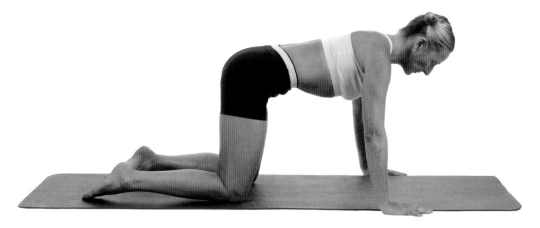

2 Exhale and engage your abdominal muscles, then bend your elbows to lower your chest toward the floor, keeping your pelvis and spine neutral. The angles at your elbows should be roughly right angles.

3 Inhale to push up and straighten your arms again. Repeat 4 to 10 times.

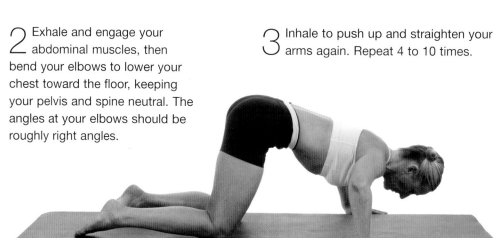

- Make sure you aren't sticking your bottom up and that you're maintaining neutral.
- Don't go any lower than the back in line with the elbows.
- Your head is in line with your spine—don't let it drop down.
- Keep thinking of pushing the floor away to engage the shoulder stabilizers.

progression—three-quarter press-up

When you've mastered the Press-Up opposite, you can make it harder by moving your knees further back from your center of gravity. Keep your shoulders in the same position as before, but take the knees back as far as you can while still keeping the pelvis neutral. Follow the directions, breathing, and awareness advice above.

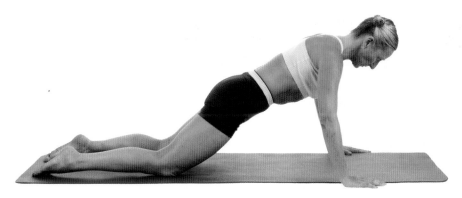

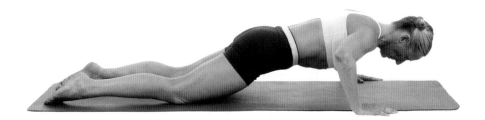

butt squeeze with press

extension   butt squeeze and upper back press (see pages 80 & 58) are preparations for this exercise

Combining these two fabulous exercises gives your power house muscles a real workout and you'll feel a great sense of length in your body as you do the movements.

1 Lie face down in the Prone Position (see page 36) and place a small pillow between your thighs. Your toes should be pointing toward each other and your heels apart. Touch your fingers together, and rest your forehead on your thumbs. Maintain neutral by engaging navel to spine, sending your pubic bone to the floor. Inhale, and imagine you can slide a $5 bill under your navel.

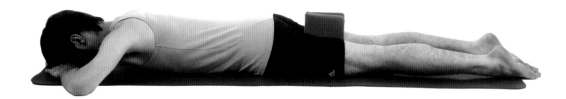

awareness

■ If you feel this working in your lower back, you may be gripping too hard with your buttock muscles. Focus on the lower abdominals working to keep your pelvis in neutral. Place a pillow under your stomach if this helps.
■ Focus on length from the crown of the head to the toes and keep lengthening, keep engaging.

2 Exhale, keep your abdominals engaged and draw your shoulderblades down your back. Lengthen the back of your neck, bringing your head up in line with the spine. Look down at the floor. Imagine a V shape running through your elbows and shoulderblades and narrowing at your waist. Don't move or lift the elbows—just think about them traveling toward your waist. At the same time, start to gently roll your heels toward each other, squeezing into the pillow. Think of the back of the inner thighs coming closer to each other and the butt working.

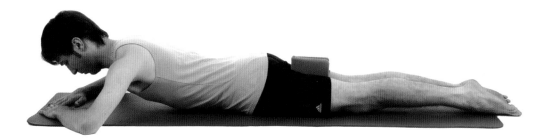

3 Inhale and maintain the position, keeping your abdominals engaged and shoulderblades down. As you progress, you will be able to hold this position for longer before releasing.

4 Repeat 6 times. When you've finished, come back to the Rest Position (see page 59). The Back Stretch (see page 43) is an alternative if you have knee problems, or you could simply roll up on your side in the fetal position.

arm circle

release/rotation   side-lying preparation (see page 81) is a preparation for this exercise

This is the ultimate tension-releasing exercise, and it's great to do at the end of your workout. It provides a gentle rotation for the spine as well as a lovely stretch for the chest and front of shoulder muscles. You will need a large pillow or a rolled-up towel.

1 Lie on your side as you did in Side-Lying Preparation (see page 81), with a pillow or rolled-up towel under your head so that your neck is supported as you roll your head. Check you are lying straight on the floor with your knees bent at a right angle. Rest your arms in front of you, palms together in line with your shoulders and fingers together. Inhale, and lengthen from the crown of your head to your tailbone.

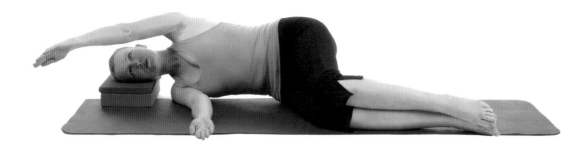

2 Exhale and engage your shoulderblades, then reach your top arm up and over your head. Let your head roll, following the movement of the arm. Maintain the distance between the top of your shoulder and your ear.

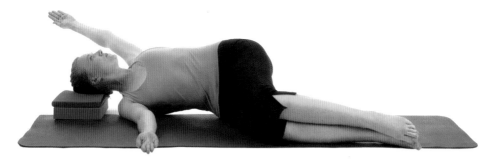

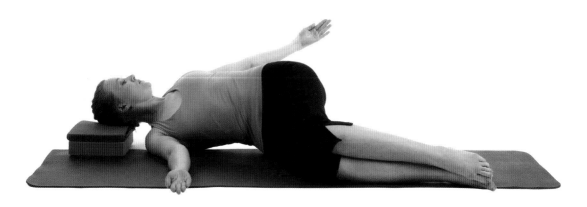

3 Breathe normally as you take the arm right round behind you. Think of sending your knees to the opposite corner of the room to stop your hips from rolling back. Bring the arm round over your hip and back to the starting position. Repeat 4 times on each side.

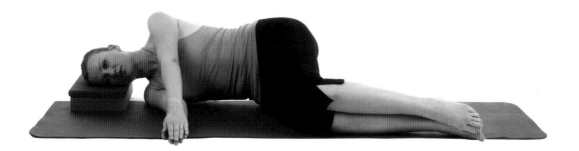

awareness

■ Think of length and energy through the arm, with your hand and wrist long.

■ Take care that your back doesn't arch by engaging your abdominals, and sending your knees away and down to the floor. Keep your waist long.

■ You can have a small pillow between your knees. This can feel more comfortable if you have a tight lower back.

■ Think of the movement coming from the waist and upper back, not the arm.

■ Make sure you roll your head with the movement, looking toward your hand as it moves around.

chapter 6

intermediate

- one leg balance
- turnout balance
- away from center

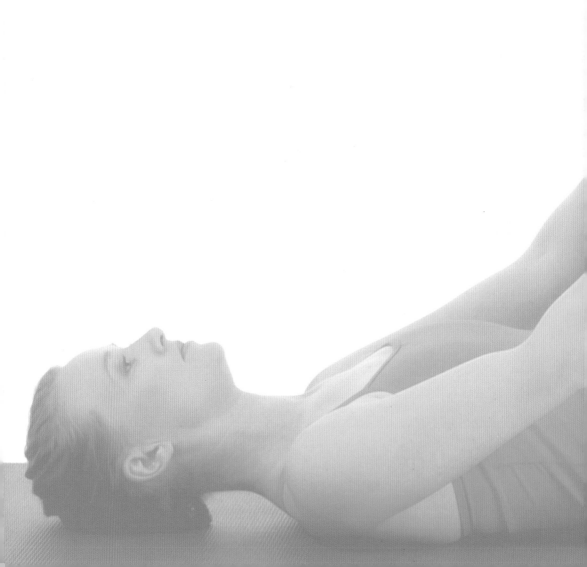

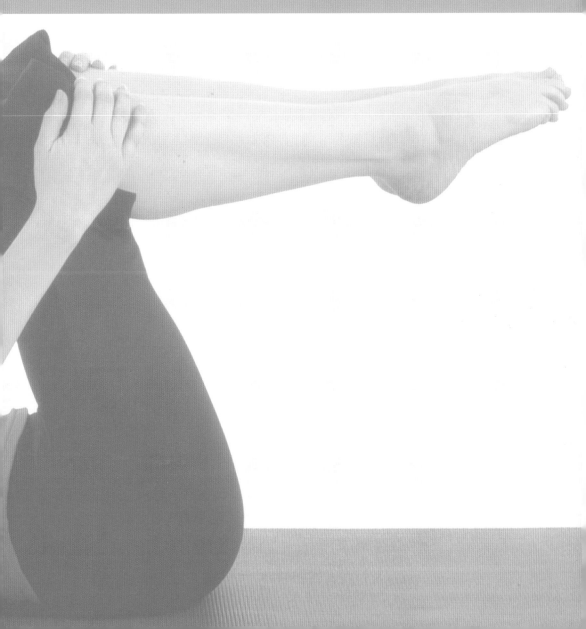

one leg balance

stability

This exercise works the glutes, or buttock muscles, as well as the muscles of the ankles and feet. If you feel your ankle or leg muscles working harder than your butt, gently tighten your butt muscles on the leg you are standing on.

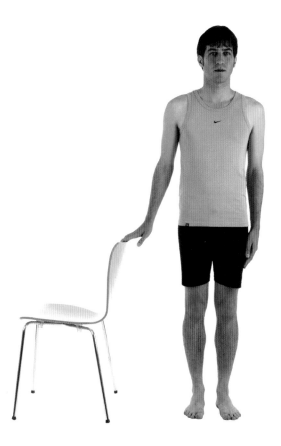

1 Stand side on to a wall or chair in a good standing posture (see page 20) and lean your hand against it for support. The leg you raise should be further away from the wall or chair—in this case, we're starting with the left leg. Inhale and lengthen the crown of the head up as the shoulderblades draw down.

progression—on toes

1 Follow steps 1 and 2, then inhale and rise up on to the ball of your right foot, making sure your weight is spread evenly across all of your toes. Hold this position, breathing normally, for about 10 seconds.
2 Exhale as you lengthen the right heel back to the floor. Build up to 4 repetitions with each leg.
3 To make this exercise harder still, try moving away from the wall a little so it is providing less support.

awareness

■ Imagine your spine being stretched like a piece of elastic—it keeps getting longer as you transfer your weight on to one leg.
■ Make sure you don't sink down into the hips at any part of the movement. Keep lengthening out of your waist.

progression—without hands

Try to do this without your hand resting on the wall or chair. Don't worry if you wobble a little—it's a sign you are working your balance reflexes. Once you can stand on one leg without holding on, challenge your balance more by trying the following: Close one eye. Close both eyes. Close both eyes and float up your arms. Try all of these while balancing on a thick rug, carpet, or slightly uneven surface—as long as you are safe.

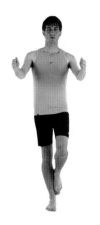

2 Exhale, engage your abdominals, and think of lifting up out of your waist as you float up your left knee bringing the side of your left foot to the calf of the right leg, with your knee pointing forward. Try to avoid leaning to one side—aim to keep your hip bones level and facing forward. Hold this position breathing normally for about 10 seconds.

3 Lower your left leg, turn around, and repeat steps 1 and 2 with your right leg raised.

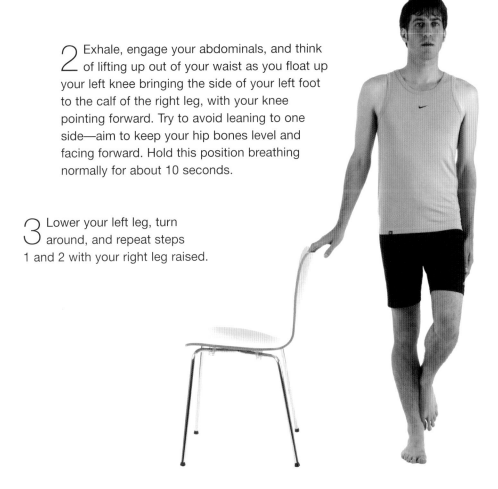

turnout balance

stability

With this exercise, you will really feel your power house muscles working. Try the progression as well, to develop a higher level of coordination. Read the awareness notes before doing this if you suffer from sciatica or lower back problems.

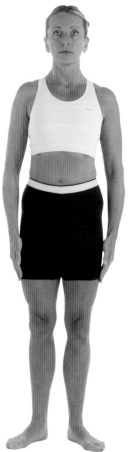

1 Stand in a good posture with your feet in a turned out position, heels toward each other and toes apart. Inhale and think of the backs of the inner thighs squeezing together—remember we talked about the muscles wrapping around your thighs (see page 37).

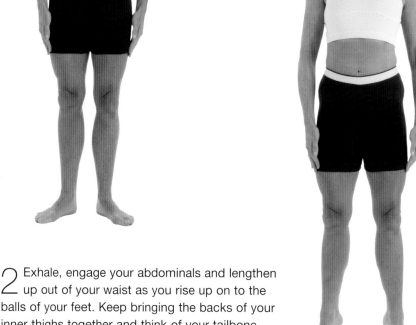

2 Exhale, engage your abdominals and lengthen up out of your waist as you rise up on to the balls of your feet. Keep bringing the backs of your inner thighs together and think of your tailbone long and pointing down.

3 Inhale to lower the heels down again, still keeping length in your spine.

4 Repeat this sequence 4 to 8 times without pausing, exhaling to rise up and inhaling to lower down. When you've finished, do a Back Stretch (see page 43).

awareness

■ If you have tight lower back muscles, the turnout position can feed back into the lower back muscles and sacroiliac area (where your spine meets your pelvis). If this is the case, do this exercise with your feet parallel or just in a slight turnout with your heels further apart.

■ Where is your weight balanced? Do you feel it more in your big toes than the other toes? Aim to spread your weight evenly across your feet.

progression—floating arms

Once you have mastered this, float up your arms in front of you (see page 64) while you are lifting and lowering with your legs (a). Alternate the arm movements. Float your right arm up while you are lifting, and lower your left arm to your side (b). Float your left arm up while you are lowering and bring your right arm back to your side.

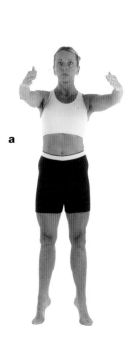

a

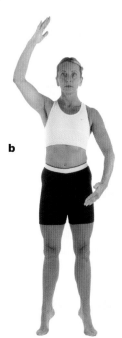

b

away from center

stability/release   knee drop (see page 48) is a preparation for this exercise

This is a real test of coordination and core stability. You will need all your powers of concentration to keep your hip bones horizontal as your limbs move out to the sides. This exercise is a good alternative to Curl-Up if you have neck problems.

1 Lie on your back in the Relaxation Position (see page 16) and raise your arms in line with your shoulders. Inhale to lengthen and draw your shoulderblades down.

2 Exhale, engage your abdominals, and lower your right knee to the side as you take your left arm out to the floor level with your shoulder.

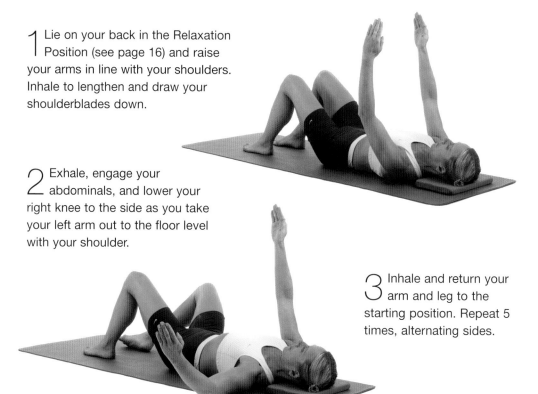

3 Inhale and return your arm and leg to the starting position. Repeat 5 times, alternating sides.

awareness

- There will be a tendency for the arm and leg which are not working to try and counterbalance the movement by moving in the opposite direction. To keep them still, you will need to focus on keeping the back of the neck long, shoulderblades down, pelvis and spine neutral, abdominals engaged, and ribs softened downward.
- Think of your ribs and hips moving toward each other, to prevent the ribs opening up.
- Concentrate on keeping your pelvis level and completely still, only dropping the knee out as far as you can while keeping the pelvis stable.

variation 1

1 When you have completed the last exercise, remain in the starting position with your knees bent and feet on the floor, and your arms in the air in line with your shoulders (a).
2 Exhale and take your left arm out to the floor at shoulder level, while rolling your head to the right. This might be easier without a pillow under your head. Let your head sink down and release your jaw. Repeat 4 or 5 times on each side, alternating sides (b).

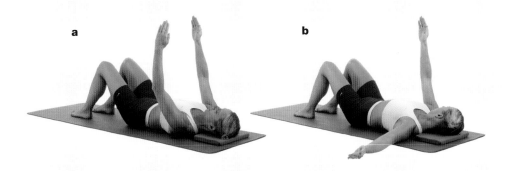

a   **b**

variation 2

1 Lie in the Relaxation Position and bring your knees up one at a time so that they are at right angles to your hips, with your big toes touching and your shins parallel to the floor. Raise your arms but keep your palms facing away. Inhale and think about creating length between your shoulders and your ears (a).
2 Exhale, engage your abdominals and lower your right foot, keeping the knee bent. Tap on the floor with your toes, and at the same time take your left arm to the side of your head. Take it down as far as you can while maintaining a neutral pelvis and keeping your ribs softened downward. Avoid taking your arm so far back that you arch your back (b).
3 Inhale to return to the starting position. Repeat 4 times on each side.

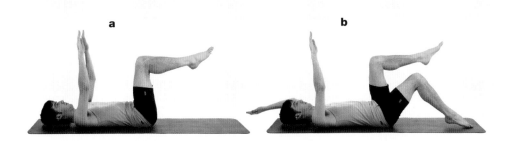

a   **b**

the hundred—with long legs

flexion/stability   the hundred (see pages 74 & 98) is a preparation for this exercise

This version of The Hundred requires more abdominal strength because the legs are straightened. If you have tight hamstrings, you may need to stretch them first (see page 72). If necessary, keep your legs slightly bent.

1 Lie on your back in the Relaxation Position (see page 16). Engage your abdominals and float your knees up one at a time so that they are at right angles to your hips, with your big toes touching and your shins parallel to the floor. Inhale and nod your head (see page 53).

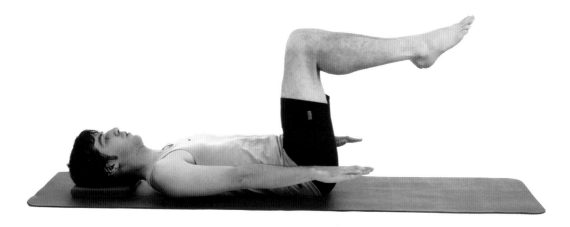

2 Exhale and curl your upper body off the floor, looking toward your navel. Keep your abdominals engaged, and think about your chest and back sinking into the mat.

awareness

■ Keep your lower back into the mat by scooping your abdominals, squeezing the backs of the inner thighs together, and tightening your buttock muscles.
■ Keep curled up high and looking at your navel.

3 Straighten your legs up toward the ceiling, squeezing the backs of the inner thighs together, with your toes softly pointing. Pump your arms up and down, thinking of the movement coming from the muscles of your upper back. Breathe in through your nose 5 times then breathe out through your mouth 5 times. Keep looking at your navel, so that your neck muscles don't overwork.

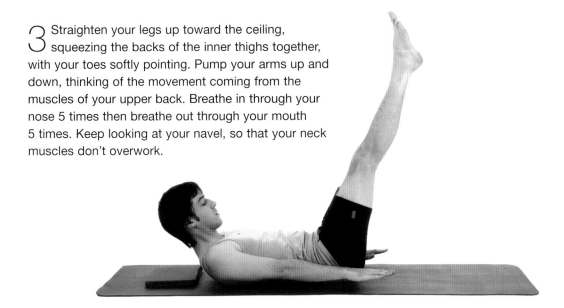

4 After 100, or as many as you can do, bend your knees to your chest and lower your upper body to the floor. Bring your legs down one at a time.

progression—legs lowered

This is an exercise from Joseph Pilates' Classic Mat sequence. Don't attempt it if you experienced any back discomfort in the last version.

1 Follow steps 1, 2, and 3 above, then lower your legs until they are at an angle of 45° from the ground. Lower your legs to the degree that you can maintain while still keeping your back pressed into the mat, with your navel engaged to the spine.
2 Pump your arms and breathe, as in step 3 above.
3 Come down by bending your knees to your chest, then rolling your upper body and head down to the floor.

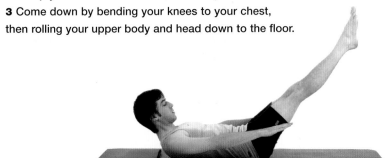

single leg stretch

flexion　single leg preparation (see page 100) is a preparation for this exercise

This is another exercise from the Classic Mat series, and it utilizes all the principles of Pilates. It will strengthen your abdominal core as well as providing a good stretch for the hamstrings and hip flexors.

1 Lie on your back in the Relaxation Position (see page 16). Clasp your hands behind your head to support it, with your elbows open just in front of your ears. Exhale, engage your abdominals and float your knees up one at a time, so that they are at right angles to your hips, with your big toes touching and your shins parallel to the floor. Inhale and nod your head, thinking of lengthening your spine.

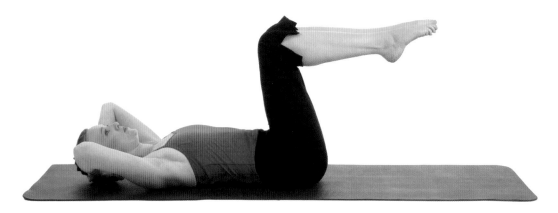

2 Exhale, engage the abdominals, then curl your upper body off the mat, looking toward your navel.

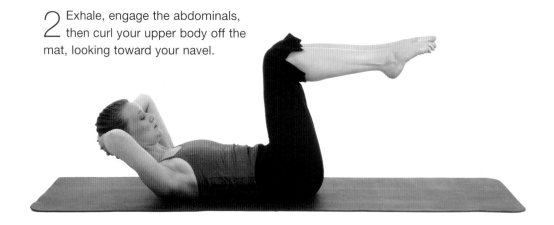

3 Inhale, keeping your abdominals engaged, ribs softened downward, and shoulderblades drawn down.

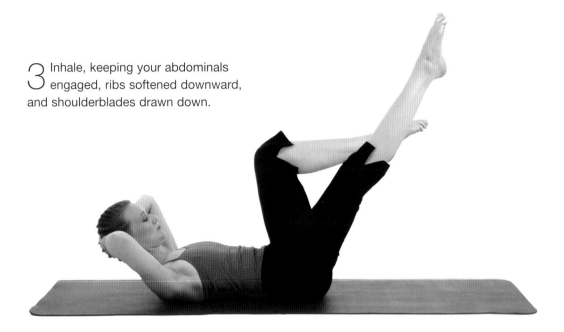

4 Exhale and straighten your right leg away, with the foot softly pointed.

5 Inhale to return the right leg. Exhale to lengthen the left. Repeat 6 times with each leg, then lower your legs to the floor, one at a time.

awareness

■ Make sure you don't roll to one side as you straighten your leg—keep both sides of the waist long.

■ If you feel any discomfort in the lower back, try one of the following adjustments: Place a small, flat pillow or folded hand towel under your hips; bring the bent knee closer to your chest; or keep the leg that is straightening higher off the floor. Or try all three to see what works for you.

■ If you have short hamstrings, you may have to do this exercise with a slightly bent leg until you are more flexible.

■ If you have neck problems, leave your head down, use a bigger pillow, and straighten your legs upward rather than away from you in step 4.

leg stretch with arms

This requires a further level of coordination as it introduces arm movements to the Single Leg Stretch (see page 126).

1 Lie on your back in the Relaxation Position (see page 16). Exhale, engage your abdominals and float your knees up one at a time, so that they are at right angles to your hips and your shins are parallel to the floor. Your knees are apart, with your big toes touching, and your feet are softly pointed. Place your right hand on the outside of your right knee. Place your left hand on the inside of your right knee, keeping the elbows open. Inhale, draw your shoulderblades down, and nod your head.

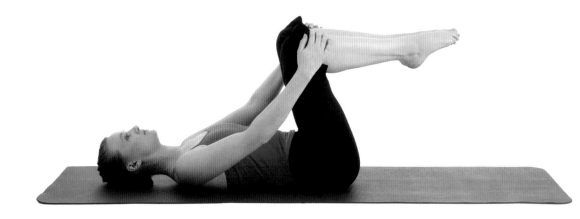

awareness

■ If you feel any discomfort in your neck, try supporting your head with your arms, or leave your head on the floor supported by a large pillow, and just move your legs.

2 Exhale, engage your abdominals, soften your ribs down, and curl your upper body off the mat. At the same time, straighten your left leg away, as you did in Single Leg Stretch (see page 126), and slide your right hand down your right calf.

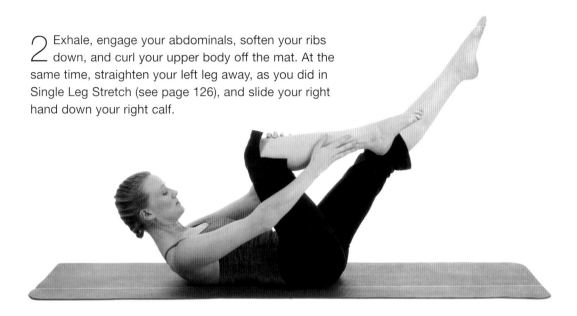

3 Inhale and bend your left leg back again, and move your hands to your left leg.

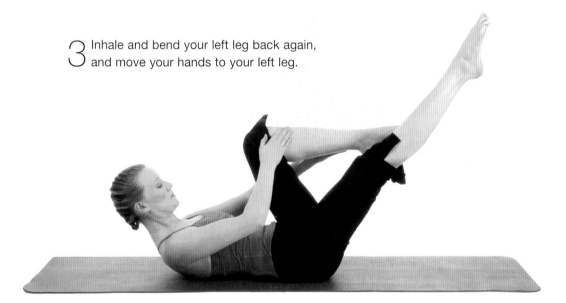

4 Exhale to straighten the right leg. Repeat 8 times for each leg, alternating legs.

double leg stretch

flexion

The aim of this exercise is to strengthen the abdominals and deep neck flexors, and to coordinate breathing with movement. It is a good stretch for the hamstrings but if your hamstrings are tight, do some Hamstring Stretches (see page 72) before you start.

1 Lie on your back in the Relaxation Position (see page 16). Exhale, engage your abdominals and float your knees up one at a time, so that they are at right angles to your hips and your shins are parallel to the floor. Your knees are apart and your feet are softly pointed with the big toes touching. Clasp your hands behind your head to support it, elbows wide and chest open. Inhale to lengthen through your spine.

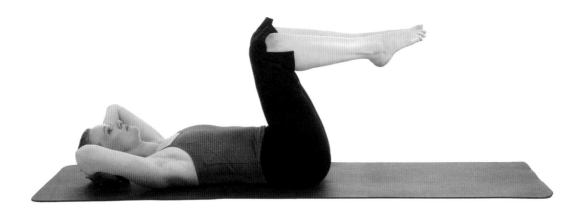

awareness

■ If your hamstrings are tight, this may pull on your lower back as you straighten your legs. Try the modifications suggested for the Single Leg Stretch (see page 127).
■ Keep your head heavy in your hands, but make sure you are not pulling on the neck.
■ The further you take your legs away from your body, the harder your abdominals have to work to keep your pelvis in neutral. If your lower back arches, bring your legs closer to your body—don't let them fall away from you. You may decide to keep your knees bent a little, depending on the length of your hamstrings.
■ If you experience neck discomfort, make sure your eyes are directed toward your navel or pubic bone.

2 Exhale, engage your abdominals and curl your upper body up from the mat, at the same time straightening both legs. Squeeze the backs of the inner thighs together, looking toward your navel.

3 Inhale, maintaining the distance between the tops of your shoulders and your ears.

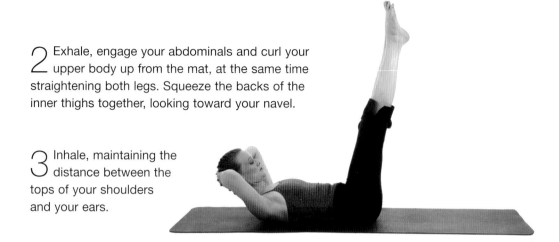

4 Exhale and curl your upper body down—think of it lengthening away—and bend your knees back to the starting position. Repeat 6 to 8 times.

progression—with arms

In this progression, the leg action is coordinated with bringing your arms to your sides—as in The Hundred (see page 124) but without the pumping action.

1 Adopt the starting position in step 1 opposite, but place your hands on the outsides of your knees, with your elbows open and shoulderblades drawn down your back (a). Inhale to lengthen your spine, and nod your head.
2 Exhale, engage your abdominals, and curl your upper body upward. At the same time straighten your legs, squeezing the backs of the inner thighs together. Keep your legs slightly turned out at the hips. Bring your arms down to the sides of your body and hold them slightly off the floor (b).
3 Inhale to lower your upper body in a controlled manner, while bending your knees back to the starting position and bringing your hands back to the outsides of your knees. Repeat 6 to 8 times.

a

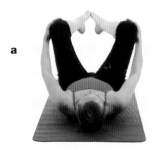

b

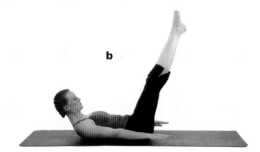

baby cobra

extension   upper back press (see page 58) is a preparation for this exercise

This exercise takes your spine to a greater level of extension, and is a lovely movement to open up the front of the body. You will be working your upper back muscles and your abdominals, while trying not to let the lower back collapse.

1 Lie on the floor in the Prone Position (see page 36) with your toes toward each other and heels apart. Extend your arms out from your shoulders and bend them so that your elbows are bent and your forearms are roughly at right angles to your elbows. Rest your forehead on the floor, or on a small paperback book. Maintain neutral by engaging your navel toward your spine and sending your pubic bone to the floor. Inhale and feel the spine lengthen.

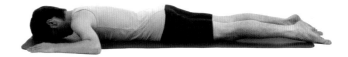

2 Exhale and draw your shoulderblades down your back. Draw the backs of your inner thighs together. Think of pressing the floor away with your elbows. Lift your upper body slowly up off the floor, keeping your ribs and breastbone down for as long as you can. Only come up as far as you can maintain neutral.

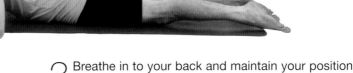

3 Breathe in to your back and maintain your position. Exhale to slowly lengthen back down to the mat. When you've finished, do a stretch in the Rest Position (see page 59).

awareness

■ Take care not to shorten at the back of the neck or to come up so high that you compress the lower back. Listen to your body and focus on the places where you feel the exercise working.

seated side reach

stability

The challenge here is to keep a neutral position while sitting, and to stabilize the shoulderblades. It's best if you can find a stretch band for this—a stretchy scarf or a pair of pantyhose won't work as well.

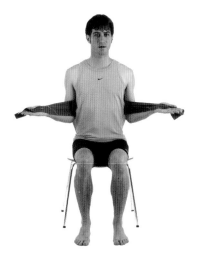

1 Sit on a chair in a good sitting position (see page 22) with your feet firmly on the floor in line with your hips. Place the band around your upper mid back and hold it under your thumbs in front, with your elbows bent at the sides of the body. Your palms are facing forward, fingers long. The tighter the band is stretched, the harder this exercise will be, because you'll be working against more resistance. Inhale, lengthen the crown of your head to the ceiling, and feel your shoulderblades draw down your back.

2 Exhale, engage your abdominals and reach your arms straight out to the sides, stretching the band. Keep your shoulderblades down and fingers long.

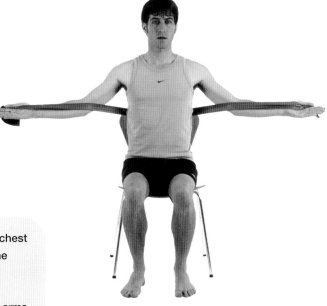

awareness

■ Make sure you don't stick your chest out or arch your back—think of the tailbone dropping behind you.
■ Visualize width across your collarbones as you straighten your arms.
■ Keeping thinking of lengthening up through the crown of the head as the shoulderblades draw down your back.

3 Inhale, and bend your elbows back in to the sides of your body. Repeat the exercise 4 to 6 times.

side reach and rotation

| rotation | seated rotation (see page 106) is a preparation for this exercise |

This exercise adds the resistance of the stretch band to develop the rotation exercises from Starting Off and Moving On. Most people use their necks rather than initiating the movement from their trunks, unless their neck is stiff, in which case they turn their whole body.

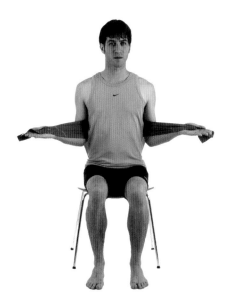

1 Sit on a chair in a good sitting position (see page 22) with your feet firmly on the floor in line with your hips. Place the band around your upper mid back and hold it under your thumbs in front, with your elbows bent at the sides of the body. Your palms are facing away from you, fingers long. The tighter the band is stretched, the harder this exercise will be. Inhale, lengthen the crown of your head to the ceiling, and feel your shoulderblades draw down your back.

awareness

- You will probably find it easier to turn to one side than the other. The key is to keep the weight on your sitting bones and buttocks even on both sides.
- Make sure your knees stay level—don't cheat and let one knee move forward.
- Keep your hip bones level and your pelvis in neutral.
- Keep both arms stretched out to the sides—don't let the opposite arm start to follow round to the side you are rotating toward, as in the photograph on the right. Keep the spine long, and shoulders down away from the ears.

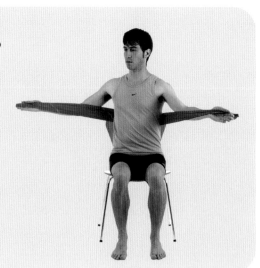

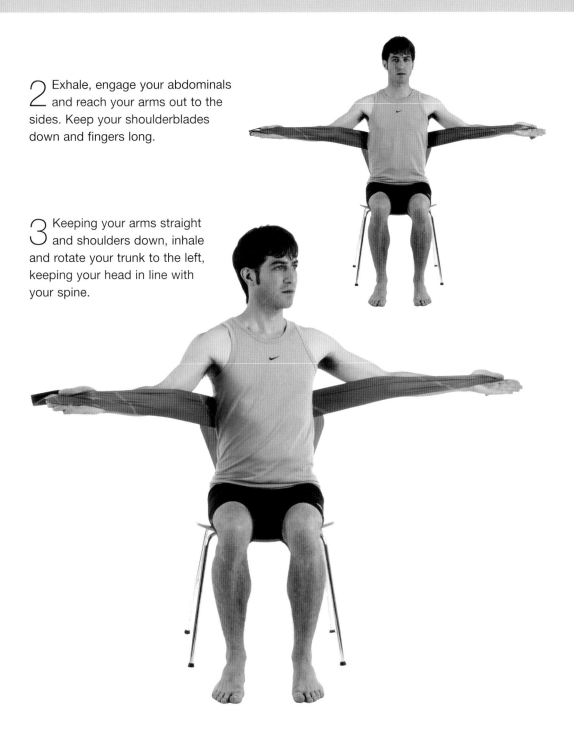

2 Exhale, engage your abdominals and reach your arms out to the sides. Keep your shoulderblades down and fingers long.

3 Keeping your arms straight and shoulders down, inhale and rotate your trunk to the left, keeping your head in line with your spine.

4 Exhale and turn back to the center, still keeping your arms straight. Inhale as you bend your elbows back to your sides, keeping your shoulders down.

5 Repeat, turning to the right in step 3, then do 2 or 4 repetitions on each side, keeping your spine long.

single leg kick

extension/stability

In this exercise, you will be stabilizing to keep a neutral spine, testing your power house muscles, and building your coordination skills. It's a good exercise for keeping the kneecaps in good alignment, but if you have a knee injury seek advice from a physician before trying it.

1 You will be breathing normally throughout this exercise. Lie in the Prone Position (see page 36), and rest your head on your folded hands. Keep your upper body relaxed and wide, your pubic bone down into the mat, and your legs together with your big toes touching each other.

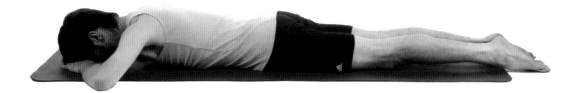

2 Engage navel to spine and squeeze the backs of the inner thighs together and engage your buttock muscles. Kick your right foot up to your buttocks, in two small pulses.

awareness

- Keep drawing your shoulders down your back and do not allow the lower back to hollow. If you feel this exercise in your lower back, keep your upper body on the floor and just do the leg action.
- Once you are familiar with the movement, do a body scan: Shoulders down, chest and abdominals lifted, pubic bone down, inner thighs and buttocks squeezing.
- Keep your hips level and your pelvis still as you move your legs.
- Think of squeezing the inner thighs together, as if your muscles are wrapping around from the front of the inner thighs to the back, while your inner thighs and knees are stuck together with glue.

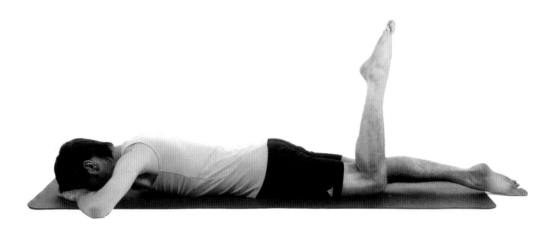

3 As you are straightening your right leg down, kick your left leg up two pulses so that the legs pass each other in mid air. If you can, don't let the straight leg touch the floor in between kicks. Repeat 4 to 6 times with each leg.

progression—heel kicks in sphinx position

1 You will be breathing normally throughout this exercise. Lie in the Prone Position and bend your elbows in line with your shoulders. You can make a fist with your hands or rest your palms down on the floor. Keep your pubic bone down into the mat, and your legs together with your big toes touching each other.

2 Engage your abdominals and think of pressing your elbows into the floor to lift your chest. This helps to make your shoulderblades draw down your back and away from your ears. Squeeze your buttock muscles and the backs of your inner thighs together.

3 Kick your right foot to your buttocks, with two small pulses. As you are straightening your right leg, kick your left leg up for two pulses, so that the legs pass each other in mid air. Try not to let the straight leg touch the floor in between kicks. Keep lifting the abdominals away from the floor. Repeat 4 to 6 times with each leg.

the v stretch

stability

This is a lovely, re-energizing stretch, which is especially good for the backs of the legs. It's nice to finish with a stretch in the Rest Position (see page 59) afterward.

1 Kneel on all fours in the Four Point Kneeling Position (see page 25), with your toes tucked under. Inhale, press the ground away, and lengthen the spine.

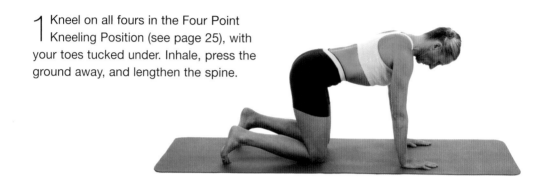

2 Exhale, engage your abdominals, and lift both your knees about 2 inches off the mat, pressing into your toes and your hands. Keep your pelvis neutral.

3 Inhale to maintain the position, still pushing the ground away.

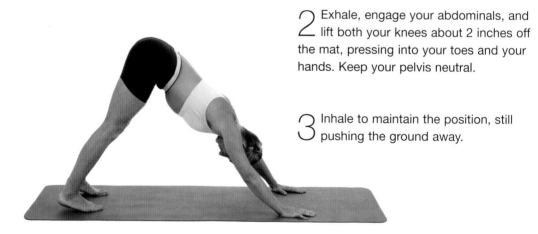

awareness

■ Make sure that your weight is evenly distributed across the heels of the hands and all of your fingers. Cup your hand a little if it helps.

4 Exhale and straighten your legs so that your hips and heels are pointing up to the ceiling. Inhale, lengthening your tailbone toward the ceiling.

5 Exhale as you bend your knees back to the floor. Repeat 4 times.

mermaid

stability   side bend (see page 92) is a preparation for this exercise

This gives the most amazing stretch down the sides of the body. Be sure to follow the instructions and awareness points carefully, and you'll find that it's not as complicated as it sounds.

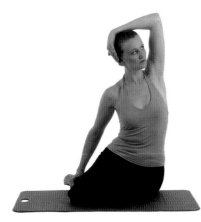

1 Sit back on your heels and drop your hips to your left side. Hold on to your right ankle with your right hand. Raise your left arm up to the ceiling and bend your elbow so that your left hand comes across to your right ear, with your left elbow pointing to the ceiling. Inhale and turn your head to the left to look into your left arm. Lift the elbow high to the ceiling, and draw your shoulderblades down your back.

2 Exhale, engage your abdominals and keep reaching your left elbow up to the ceiling, as you stretch up and over toward the right. Feel the distance between your left ribs and hip increasing as you visualize your left hip dropping toward the floor. You can pull on your right ankle a little to give opposition to the stretch—but keep your shoulders down.

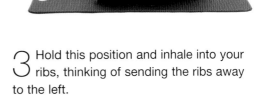

awareness

■ Keep thinking "drop shoulders," as it's easy for your shoulders to creep up to your ears in this movement.
■ As you are stretching to the side, don't let your trunk or elbow come forward. Keep your hip bones and chest facing forward.

3 Hold this position and inhale into your ribs, thinking of sending the ribs away to the left.

4 Breathe out, and come back to the starting position. Repeat 2 or 3 times on each side.

double leg lift

stability   lying side reach and shell (see pages 83 & 82) are preparations for this exercise

This side-lying position requires you to balance your weight as you raise both your upper and lower legs from the floor. It is particularly good for working the inner thigh muscles and the outer hip muscles, which are both important for pelvic stability.

1 Lie on your side with your lower arm stretched up under your head, so that it supports your head in line with your body. Draw the shoulderblades down to increase the distance between the ears and the shoulders. If this is not comfortable, bring the lower arm down so it rests in front of you, in line with the shoulders, and use a thick book or firm pillow under your head. Line yourself up so that your spine is straight. Make sure that shoulder is over shoulder, hip over hip, and both legs are straight and slightly in front of your spine. Rest the top hand on the floor in front of you.

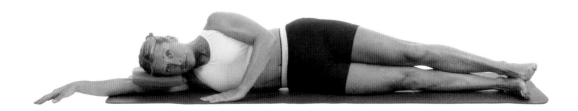

2 Inhale, engage your abdominals, and lift your top leg in line with your hip, flexing the foot. Think about the length along your spine and the length from the hip through to the heel.

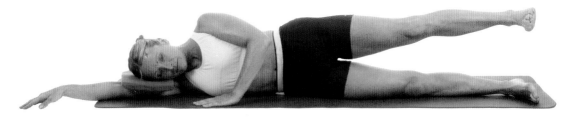

3 Exhale, keeping your abdominals engaged, and lift the lower leg to come toward or meet the top leg. Keep lengthening down the sides of the waist and legs.

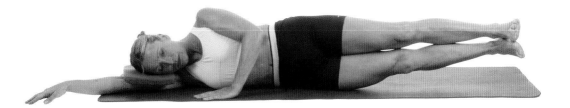

4 Inhale and slowly lower the bottom leg, then exhale as you lower the top leg. Repeat 6 to 8 times on each side.

awareness

■ Check that you are not shortening into your waist—think about the length down both sides of the waist.
■ Focus your eyes straight ahead or slightly down.
■ If you need to, you can do this exercise with a pillow between your head and arm so your head is supported in correct alignment. Keep length between the shoulder and the ear.
■ Lift your top leg so that it is in line with the hip, but no higher.

four point to plank

| stability | press-up and leg slide (see pages 110 & 75) are preparations for this exercise |

You need a very strong center for this exercise. It is a real challenge to your ability to keep your pelvis level as you take the second leg out. If you feel you are not ready for this, keep practicing the V stretch (see page 138) instead.

1 Kneel on all fours in the Four Point Kneeling Position (see page 25). Inhale and press the ground away, lengthening your shoulders away from your ears.

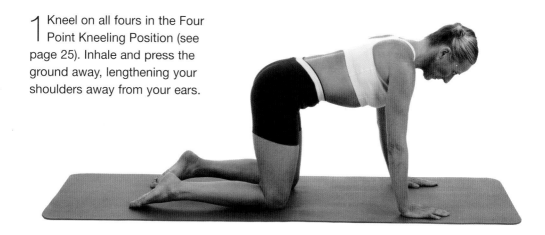

2 Exhale, engage your abdominals, and slide the right leg away until it is straight. Tuck the toes under, thinking of lengthening the heel away.

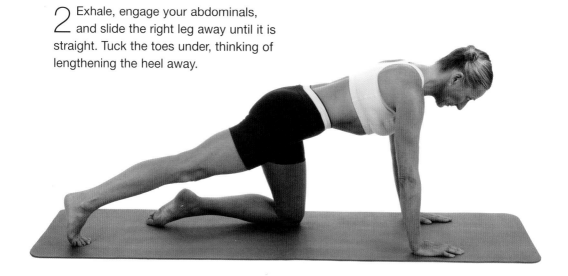

3 Inhale, and hold the position, keeping a strong center.

4 Exhale and take your weight onto your right leg as you straighten your left leg beside it, keeping your feet hip distance apart. Keep lifting your navel away from the floor, shoulderblades drawn down and hips absolutely level. Inhale and maintain this position.

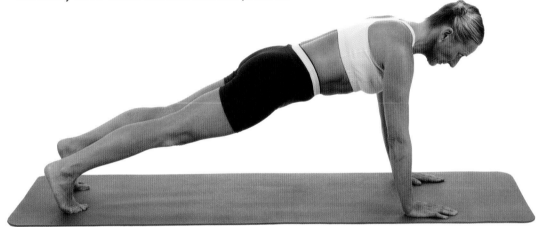

5 Exhale and slide your right leg back, without letting your lower back sag. Keep your shoulders away from your ears and your head in line with your spine. Inhale and hold.

6 Exhale, and return your left leg in the same way, still keeping your abdominals engaged.

awareness

■ Be careful that your head doesn't hang down or your lower back dip when you have both legs out.
■ Keep your legs hip distance apart throughout, with your hip bones facing the floor and abdominals firmly engaged.
■ Avoid locking your elbows at any stage.
■ Think of the ear, shoulder, and hip being in line.

chapter 7

programs

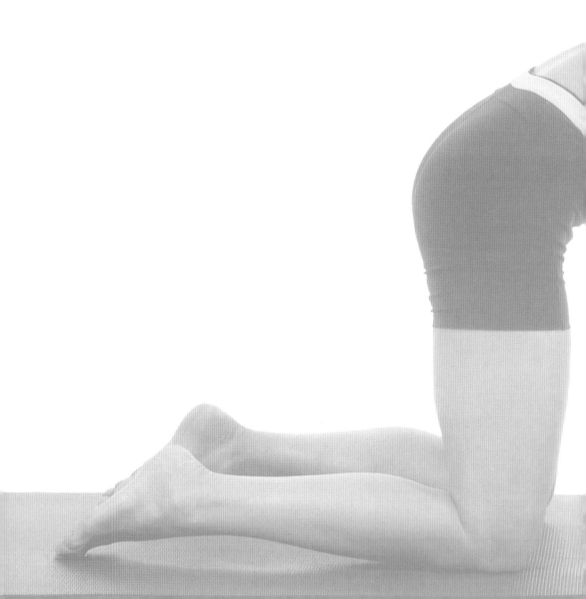

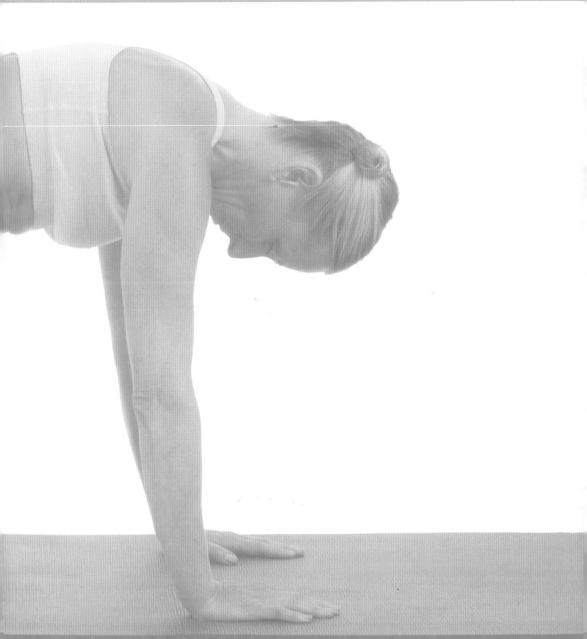

starting off sequence

This group of exercises will give you a good balanced workout. Adjust the number of repetitions, depending on how much time you have available. Check back and read the instructions and awareness points to ensure correct technique. Keep thinking about maintaining the length of your spine and perform the exercises at a slow controlled pace.

25 minutes

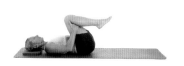

Back stretch
(see page 43)

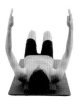

Shoulder drop
(see page 44)

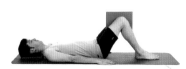

Inner thigh squeeze
(see page 66)

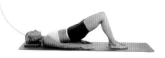

Spine curl—with or without arms
(see page 50)

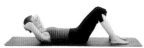

Curl-up
(see page 54)

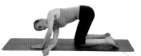

Folding through
(see page 56)

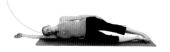

Lying side reach
(see page 83)

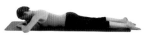

Upper back press
(see page 58)

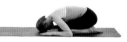

Rest position
(see page 59)

45–60 minutes

Balancing
(see page 62)

Floating up arms
(see page 64)

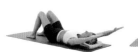

Shoulder release
(see page 68)

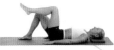

Single knee fold
(see page 70)

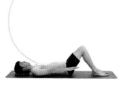

The hundred—
preparation
(see page 74)

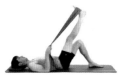

Hamstring stretch
(see page 72)

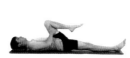

Hip flexor stretch
(see page 73)

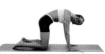

Cat
(see page 76)

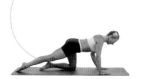

Four point leg slide
(see page 75)

Chair roll-down
(see page 77)

Seated side bend
(see page 78)

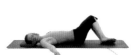

Hip roll
(see page 79)

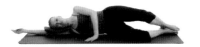

The shell
(see page 82)

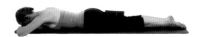

Butt squeeze
(see page 80)

moving on sequence

Once you have mastered the exercises in the Warm-Up and Starting Off, familiarize yourself with the exercises in Moving On. As with Starting Off, you can vary the number of repetitions depending on how much time you have. The programs are designed to include a warm-up but if there are other Warm-Up exercises you prefer, do them first.

Work at a comfortable pace, aiming for good alignment and abdominal control. If an exercise doesn't feel comfortable, look back at the instructions to see if there are any variations you could do.

25 minutes

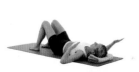

Shoulder release
(see page 68)

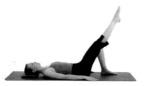

Single leg preparation
(see page 100)

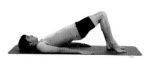

Spine curl with heel lift
(see page 96)

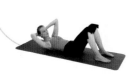

Oblique curl-up
(see page 102)

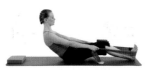

Roll back with band
(see page 104)

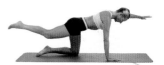

Opposite arm and leg lift
(see page 108)

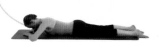

Upper back press
(see page 58)

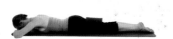

Butt squeeze
(see page 80)

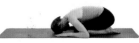

Rest position
(see page 59)

45–60 minutes

Standing roll-down
(see page 86)

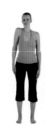

Shoulder roll
(see page 88)

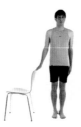

Balancing
(see page 62)

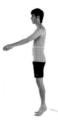

Balance and
float arms
(see page 90)

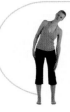

Side bend
(see page 92)

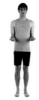

Arm opening
(see page 89)

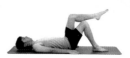

Double knee fold
(see page 94)

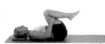

Back stretch
(see page 43)

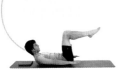

The hundred—
with abdominals
(see page 98)

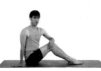

Seated rotation
(see page 106)

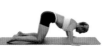

Press-up
(see page 110)

Upper back press
(see page 58)

Butt squeeze
(see page 80)

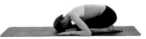

Rest position
(see page 59)

intermediate sequence

Intermediate exercises should only be attempted once you have worked through Starting Off and Moving On, as many of the exercises in the earlier stages are preparations for the strength and flexibility you will require at this stage. Always re-read the awareness points. If any movement feels uncomfortable, either do an easier variation or choose another exercise that feels good for you. Keep focused and centered on your workout, giving yourself time and being patient. Do 4 to 6 repetitions of each of the following:

25 minutes

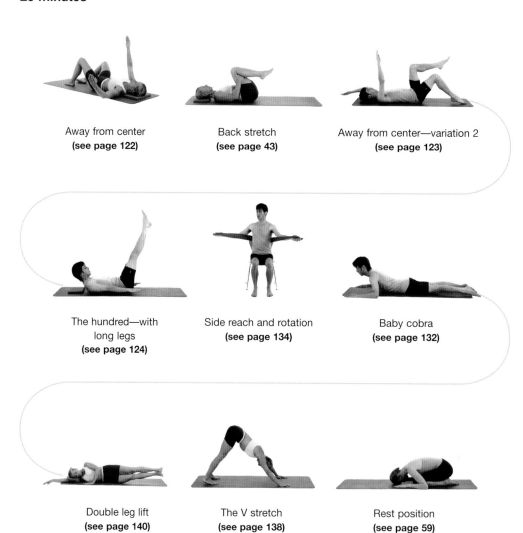

Away from center
(see page 122)

Back stretch
(see page 43)

Away from center—variation 2
(see page 123)

The hundred—with
long legs
(see page 124)

Side reach and rotation
(see page 134)

Baby cobra
(see page 132)

Double leg lift
(see page 140)

The V stretch
(see page 138)

Rest position
(see page 59)

45–60 minutes

Standing roll-down
(see page 86)

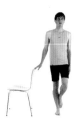

One leg balance
(see page 118)

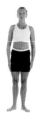

Turnout balance
(see page 120)

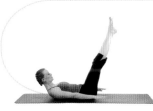

Roll back to floor
(see page 105)

Shoulder release
(see page 68)

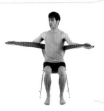

Single leg stretch
(see page 126)

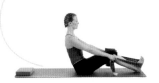

Double leg stretch
(see page 130)

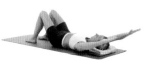

Mermaid
(see page 139)

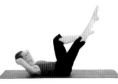

Side reach
and rotation
(see page 134)

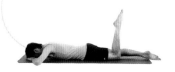

Single leg kick
(see page 136)

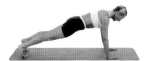

Four point to plank
(see page 142)

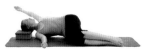

Arm circle
(see page 114)

flowing sequence

In this sequence, all the movements flow well from one to the next. You'll go from standing to all fours, to lying on your back, then lying on your front, lying on your side, and back up to standing again. It encompasses movements from all of the stages, so don't try it until you are familiar with all of these exercises. Just do 1 or 2 repetitions of each move.

15 minutes

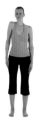 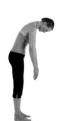 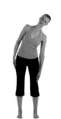 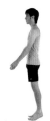

Shoulder roll	Standing roll-down	Standing side bend	Balance and float arms
(see page 88)	**(see page 86)**	**(see page 92)**	**(see page 90)**

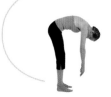 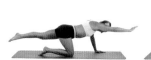 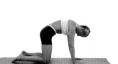

Standing roll-down	Opposite arm and leg lift	The cat	Mermaid—to left
(see page 86)	**(see page 108)**	**(see page 76)**	**(see page 139)**

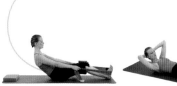 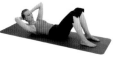 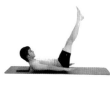 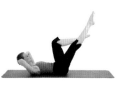

Roll back with band	Oblique curl-up	The hundred—with long legs	Single leg stretch
(see page 104)	**(see page 102)**	**(see page 124)**	**(see page 126)**

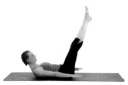

Double leg stretch
(see page 130)

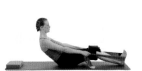

Roll back with band
(see page 104)

Mermaid—right side
(see page 139)

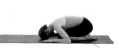

Rest position
(see page 59)

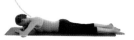

Upper back press
(see page 58)

Butt squeeze
(see page 80)

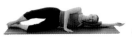

The shell—right side
(see page 82)

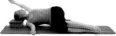

Arm circle
(see page 114)

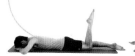

Single leg kick
(see page 136)

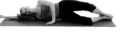

The shell—left side
(see page 82)

Arm circle
(see page 114)

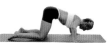

Press-up
(see page 110)

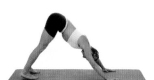

The V stretch
(see page 138)

Standing roll-down
(see page 86)

everyday pilates

For Pilates to be effective, it has to be incorporated into your everyday life. Try to transfer the good movement and posture habits you have learned in the exercises into your day-to-day activities.

Everyday Pilates is not a substitute for your regular sessions, because you won't be using the same level of concentration that you apply to your workouts. However, everyday Pilates is a useful complement to your more focused practice sessions. Practice Active Standing and Sitting (see pages 37–38) whenever you can—while cooking, driving, shopping, talking on the phone, cleaning your teeth, waiting for a bath to run, standing in line at the supermarket check-out, or waiting for a physician's or dentist's appointment.

If you spend most of your day sitting, you can practice the sitting routine below without leaving your desk—it only takes a few minutes. Why not stand up to take telephone calls and practice Active Standing? Give yourself a break from sitting whenever you can. Do the standing routine when you have a few spare minutes at home, to help improve lower body circulation.

sitting at your desk

5 minutes

Chair roll-down
(see page 77)

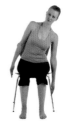

Seated side bend
(see page 78)

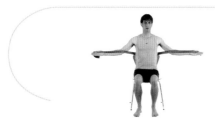

Seated side reach
(see page 133)

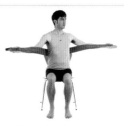

Seated side reach
and rotation
(see page 134)

standing home routine

Do this instead of sitting and watching TV, or while you are waiting for dinner to cook, or for the bath to run—or whenever you think of it. (If you haven't got a stretch band for the side reach and rotation, do these exercises without one.)

10–15 minutes

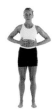

Standing and breathing
(see page 29)

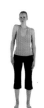

Shoulder roll
(see page 88)

Standing roll-down
(see page 86)

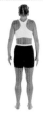

Shoulder shrug
(see page 42)

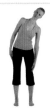

Standing side bend
(see page 92)

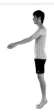

Balance and float arms
(see page 90)

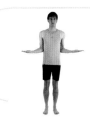

Arm opening
(see page 89)

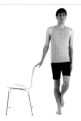

One leg balance
(see page 118)

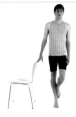

One leg balance on toes
(see page 118)

tv workout

You can do this routine in front of the TV. Use the Roll-Down as a Warm-Up, before the program you want to watch has begun, and finish with the Cat and Rest Position when the program is over.

15–20 minutes

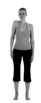
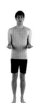
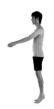

| Standing roll-down
(see page 86) | Shoulder roll
(see page 88) | Arm opening
(see page 89) | Balance and float arms
(see page 90) |

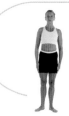

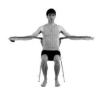
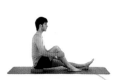

| Turnout balance
(see page 120) | One leg balance
(see page 118) | Seated side reach
(see page 133) | Sofa stretch
(see page 23) |

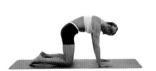
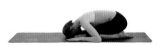

| The cat
(see page 76) | Rest position
(see page 59) |

walking or jogging

Walk whenever you can—find an excuse to use your legs instead of the car—and transfer your good Pilates standing posture into active walking sessions. Wear a good pair of walking shoes. As you walk, think of the crown of your head lengthening up, imagine your tailbone dropping down to the floor, and feel the opposition at work. Engage your power house muscles and roll through your feet as you walk, from the heel through to the balls of your feet and toes. Keep your weight evenly balanced across your feet. Let your arms swing in a natural alternate arm/leg pattern. Think of your neck long and your shoulderblades drawn down your back. Don't take large strides; if you want to walk faster, take quicker steps. If you move your arms faster, your legs will naturally follow.

relaxation and meditations

It's lovely to find some quiet time, run a hot bath, light some candles, dim the lights, and relax your mind and body. Sometimes, however, life isn't like that—but you should be able to find time for some meditation and breathing exercises in even the most hectic lifestyle. If you feel nervous or anxious, the breathing exercises are especially helpful; or try doing a body scan during train or bus journeys for instant relaxation— but set your alarm so you don't miss your stop!

complete chill out

You may want to record the relaxation script in your own voice before you begin—or read through it a couple of times and you will be surprised how much you remember. You can say it in the first person, as in "My arms are heavy," or in the second person as in "Your arms are heavy." The concept of "heaviness" is adapted from autogenic training.

Find yourself a quiet space where you won't be interrupted. Burn some aroma-therapy oils or light some scented candles, play some relaxing music, and have a blanket nearby in case you get cold. The relaxation technique below has three elements, but you don't have to do all three every time. If you find one element works for you more than the others, choose that, or adapt the sequence to fit the time you have available.

First of all, put your feet up by resting them on a chair, so that your knees and hips are bent at right angles. Let your arms rest on the floor by your sides, slightly away from your body, with the palms facing up—this helps to release the front of the shoulders and chest. Rest your head on a folded towel or firm pillow. If you have taped the script, just press play; if you are working from memory, start with your body scan, then the heaviness, and finally the lightness and breath.

body scan

Close your eyes, concentrate on your breathing, and take a deep, cleansing breath down to your stomach. Let out a sigh as you breathe out as fully as you can. Breathe in again slowly, feeling your stomach rise, and release with a sigh. Do this once more.

Now think about your feet. Notice any tension there, in your toes or ankles, or in your heels, and let it travel out through your feet and into the ground.

Now think about your legs, your calf muscles and all the muscles at the back of your legs, then the muscles on the front of the legs, and if there is any tension there, just let it go. Let it travel down your legs and out through your feet, into the ground.

Think about your hips. Do you notice any tension in the hips or thighs or lower back? Let it travel down your legs and out through your feet, into the ground.

Now focus on your fingers. If there is any tension in your fingers or hands, let it go out through your fingers into the ground.

Think about your arms and shoulders, your neck, chest, and mid back. If there is any tension there, let it travel out, down your arms, out through your fingers, and into the ground.

Now concentrate on your head and neck, your jaw muscles, and forehead. If there is any tension, just let it go—down your arms and out through your fingers, into the ground.

heaviness

Now feel the weight of your body on the mat; imagine you are sinking down into some warm soft sand. You can feel the imprint your body is making in the sand as you get heavier and heavier.

Repeat each of the following, three times each, only adding "and warm" if it's true:

"Both my arms are heavy [and warm]."

"Both my arms are heavy [and warm]."

"My arms and my legs are heavy [and warm]."

"My heart rate is calm and regular."

"My neck and shoulders are heavy."

"I feel calm."

Repeat your own choice of affirmation here, if you like.

And, as you feel the weight of your head sinking down into the floor, your neck muscles just let go, loose and limp, heavy and relaxed. Feel your jaw slightly open and the back of your tongue spread wide in your mouth. Release the muscles between your eyebrows, the frown muscles, and you sense a feeling of release and relaxation spreading through your entire body.

lightness

This stage will make you start feeling more alert again.

You start to feel a sensation of lightness spreading over your body.

You start to feel light and floaty, lightly relaxed.

Breathe in and send warming energy of the breath, loosening and softening, lightening your muscles.

Imagine you are breathing in some bright yellow energizing sunlight, and breathing out any tension.

Breathing in energizing bright, warm, healing light, sending it to your arms and legs, shoulders and neck, anywhere that you feel needs it.

Breathe out, and release.

Now, breathing in, send this energizing breath your chest muscles, shoulder muscles, feel your collarbones widening.

Breathe out and let go, let any tension go.

As you breathe in again, have a nice long stretch, sending the breath to your fingers and toes, opening your eyes.

Roll over onto your side in fetal position for a few minutes, then slowly use your arms to push you up into side sitting. Slowly rise when you are ready.

This relaxation method is a very effective method of bringing peace into your day, making your heart rate calm and regular, and relaxing you if you feel anxious or irritable.

index